FERRETS
HEALTH, HUSBANDRY AND DISEASES

FERRETS
HEALTH, HUSBANDRY AND DISEASES

Maggie Lloyd
MA, VetMB, CertLAS, MRCVS

**Blackwell
Science**

© 1999 by
Blackwell Science Ltd
Editorial Offices:
Osney Mead, Oxford OX2 0EL
25 John Street, London WC1N 2BL
23 Ainslie Place, Edinburgh EH3 6AJ
350 Main Street, Malden
   MA 02148 5018, USA
54 University Street, Carlton
   Victoria 3053, Australia
10, rue Casimir Delavigne
   75006 Paris, France

Other Editorial Offices:

Blackwell Wissenschafts-Verlag GmbH
Kurfürstendamm 57
10707 Berlin, Germany

Blackwell Science KK
MG Kodenmacho Building
7–10 Kodenmacho Nihombashi
Chuo-ku, Tokyo 104, Japan

First published 1999

Set in 11/15 pt Souvenir
by DP Photosetting, Aylesbury, Bucks
Printed and bound in Great Britain by
MPG Books Ltd, Bodmin, Cornwall

DISTRIBUTORS

Marston Book Services Ltd
PO Box 269
Abingdon
Oxon OX14 4YN
(*Orders:*   Tel: 01235 465500
            Fax: 01235 465555)

USA
Blackwell Science, Inc.
Commerce Place
350 Main Street
Malden, MA 02148 5018
(*Orders:*   Tel: 800 759 6102
            781 388 8250
            Fax: 781 388 8255)

Canada
Login Brothers Book Company
324 Saulteaux Crescent
Winnipeg, Manitoba R3J 3T2
(*Orders:*   Tel: 204 837-2987
            Fax: 204 837-3116)

Australia
Blackwell Science Pty Ltd
54 University Street
Carlton, Victoria 3053
(*Orders:*   Tel: 03 9347 0300
            Fax: 03 9347 5001)

A catalogue record for this title is available
from the British Library

ISBN 0-632-05178-7

Library of Congress
Cataloging-in-Publication Data
is available

For further information on
Blackwell Science, visit our website:
www.blackwell-science.com

CONTENTS

FOREWORD

Our knowledge of ferret diseases has expanded rapidly over the last 15 years. Much of the published literature comes from the USA and those who are familiar with it, and have heard speakers from that country, will be well aware of the divergent nature of the diseases that occur there compared with Europe. This is an extraordinary situation compared with the dog and cat where such differences do not occur, and is an important reason for having a UK-orientated text. Maggie Lloyd has written this book primarily for the European market, but discusses where the divergences occur and the probable reasons for them. Although many of these conditions have yet to be recorded in Europe, the author, nonetheless, discusses them in detail, thereby making the text relevant for veterinarians in the USA.

A small animal practice in the UK can now expect that up to 20% of its consultations will be for animals not included in the student's curriculum. Ferrets are one of these and are increasingly being presented to the clinician. The need for a comprehensive and up-to-date text is therefore very apparent. This book has been written with the practising veterinarian, laboratory worker, student and nurse in mind. The information is both practical, accessible and as complete as possible in the space available.

There are still many aspects of ferret disease which are unexplained and the author has to state in many places that the cause or reason is unknown. It is my hope that clinicians involved with and interested in ferrets will in the future investigate and record their work in these fields.

Michael Oxenham *B. Vet. Med. MRCVS*

ACKNOWLEDGEMENTS

I am indebted to Michael Oxenham for sharing both his lifetime of experience and his extensive bibliography and collection of photographs, slides and radiographs with me. Plates 7, 9, 10, 12, 13, 15, 17, 18 and 19 are reproduced with his kind permission.

Many grateful thanks are also due to Sarah for reading and commenting on what must have seemed endless pages of manuscript, and to Duncan and Caroline for caring for the ferrets.

Front cover photograph of Zac taken by Laurence Waters.

PREFACE

The ferret, *Mustela putorius furo*, belongs to the order Carnivora and is probably descended from the European polecat, *Mustela putorius*. Ferrets can interbreed with polecats, and have a similar appearance to them, although their masks are different and polecats have darker fur. Ferrets are also closely related to mink, stoats, weasels, otters and badgers, but unlike these other mustelids they are not truly feral and have been raised in captivity for centuries. References to the domestication of ferrets can be found as early as the fourth century BC. Greek authors record the use of ferrets as working pets for hunting and in the control of snakes, rabbits and rodents from the first century BC, and they are still used for this purpose in parts of Europe. Rodents have an extreme fear of ferrets, and only a few ferrets were required to remove many hundreds of rodents from large warehouses of grain stores. Ferrets have even been used to control rodent populations on board ship. Cable layers use ferrets in difficult conduits, to take through cords which are used to pull new cables. In addition, ferrets have been bred for their pelts and there is still a market for their fur, known as 'fitch'.

In recent years, ferrets have been increasingly kept as pets in Europe and North America. They have a reputation for being aggressive and difficult to handle, which is probably only true of nursing females and adult animals which have not been handled from a young age. Young ferrets respond well to frequent handling and soon become friendly, and they are surprisingly good when kept as children's pets, although like dogs or cats they can be unpredictable and care should be taken with young children.

Ferrets come in a variety of colours. The commonest ones are fitch (often referred to as polecat) (black guard hair, cream undercoat, black points), and albino, which tends to become yellow with age due to sebaceous secretions. Another colour which may be seen is cinnamon (beige guard hair, cream undercoat, no mask). They moult in the spring and autumn, corresponding with a seasonal fluctuation in weight. Typically, the summer coat is shorter and sparser, with the winter coat, consisting of a thick, soft undercoat with longer, glossy guard hairs, developing in the autumn.

Ferrets may be presented to the veterinary practitioner either simply in need of vaccinations, or with any one of a range of diseases as diverse as those seen in cats or dogs. This book is intended to be a practical guide to the management and diseases of ferrets to assist veterinary surgeons and veterinary nurses when presented with one of these curious and playful creatures.

SECTION 1
BIOLOGY AND
MANAGEMENT

1 ANATOMY

Ferrets belong to the family Mustelidae, and are closely related to mink, weasels, stoats, skunks, badgers and otters. Mustelids are considered to be among the most primitive of terrestrial carnivores, although they have many anatomical features in common with the dog and cat, particularly in their gastrointestinal and reproductive systems. Ferrets have short noses, short furry ears, very long tubular bodies, and short limbs, features which allow them to move freely in confined spaces and turn round in narrow tunnels. In the adult male, the body length may reach 50 cm, with the tail being another 15 cm.

This chapter is not intended to be a comprehensive description of the anatomy of the ferret; rather it is designed to be an aid to the interpretation of features which may be found on clinical or radiographic examination.

Skeletal system
(see Figure 1.1)

The vertebrae are large in comparison with the size of the animal and the vertebral formula is C7, T15, L5(6), S3 and Cy18. The cervical vertebrae are larger than the thoracic, allowing for the powerful musculature needed to move and control the head when capturing prey. The thorax is long, with 14 or 15 pairs of ribs: some ferrets may have 14 on one side and 15 on the other. The first 10 pairs of ribs are attached to the sternum, the remainder form the costal arch. The thoracic inlet, bounded by the first pair of ribs and the sternum, is very narrow, with the result that any anterior thoracic mass may rapidly result in dysphagia or dyspnoea. The caudal thorax is much wider, and encloses many of the abdominal organs. The sternum itself consists of eight bony sternebrae and a cartilaginous xiphoid.

The lumbar vertebrae are articulated so as to allow much dorsoventral movement with little lateral movement. The three sacral vertebrae are fused, the sacro-iliac joint being mainly between the first sacral vertebra and the ilium. The tail consists of 18 caudal vertebrae. The first three form the roof of the pelvic canal, and the second to the fifth have a ventral concavity which encloses an artery and a vein. The vertebrae become progressively smaller and featureless towards the tip of the tail.

The limbs are relatively short, and all four feet have five digits and claws with pads. The claws are not retractable, and may need regular trimming, particularly in old animals and those which are not working. The forelimb consists of humerus, ulna and radius, seven carpal bones arranged in two rows as in the dog, five metacarpals, and five digits. The first digit has two phalanges and the other digits have three. This limb is attached to the thorax by muscles at the omothoracic junction. The clavicle is a small, flattened rod which lies within the tendon of the brachiocephalicus muscle rather like that seen in the dog, and may be seen on x-ray craniomedial to the shoulder joint.

The hindlimb consists of the pelvis, femur, tibia and fibula, seven tarsal bones arranged as in the dog, five metatarsals, and digits as in the forelimb. The tibia is the longest limb bone, with the slender fibula articulating proximally with the lateral tibial condyle and distally with both the tibia and tibial tarsal bone. Two sesamoid bones may be seen within the stifle joint: the patella, which glides in the trochlear groove on the cranial surface of the distal femur, and the lateral fabella, situated on the caudal aspect of the lateral femoral condyle.

Ferrets have an os penis, which is j-shaped and can reach 4.5 cm in length. This can make urethral catheterisation difficult.

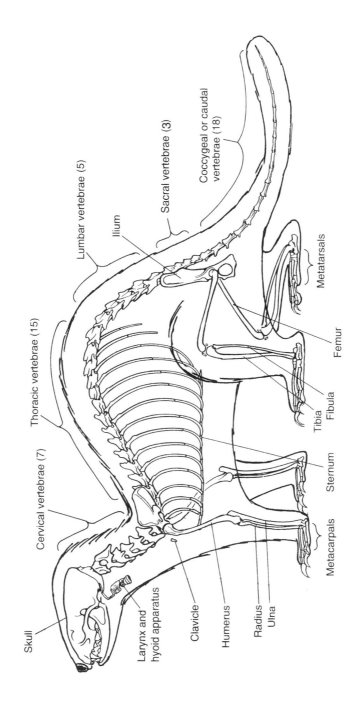

Figure 1.1 Skeleton of the ferret (adapted from An, N.Q. and Evans, H.E. 1998).

Digestive system

Ferrets have a typical carnivore digestive system. Their mouths are large: the commissures of the lips extend further caudally than the carnassial teeth and the articular fossa of the temporomandibular joint has a flange which prevents the jaw from dislocating when the mouth is opened widely. They have short, powerful jaws, which are of similar lengths, but the lower jaw is narrower than the upper jaw, allowing a shearing action when chewing. The teeth are typical of carnivores, with small incisors and long, sharp canine teeth. The upper canines may protrude beyond the lower jaw, and the roots of all the canine teeth are longer than the crowns, which is important when trying to extract them. The dental formulae are:

Deciduous dentition:

$$2\left(I\frac{4}{3} \; C\frac{1}{1} \; P\frac{3}{3}\right) = 30$$

Permanent dentition:

$$2\left(I\frac{3}{3} \; C\frac{1}{1} \; P\frac{3}{3} \; M\frac{1}{2}\right) = 34$$

At birth, there are ridges along the gums, and the deciduous teeth erupt between two and four weeks. The permanent canines appear by 47–52 days, before the deciduous canines are shed at 56–70 days. The permanent incisors erupt between six and eight weeks, and the other permanent teeth follow by ten weeks of age. It is common for ferrets to have supernumerary incisors.

The upper third premolar and lower first molar are carnassial teeth, each with three roots. All other premolars have two roots, while the upper molar has three roots and the lower second molar is tiny with only one root.

The oesophagus extends from the caudal pharynx to the cardia, and is approximately 17 to 19 cm long. The cervical region is initially dorsal to the trachea, while once it reaches the thoracic inlet it lies to the left of the trachea. The abdominal oesophagus passes through the oesophageal hiatus between the lobes of the liver to the stomach. The oesophagus has three areas of constriction: at the origin, at the point where it is crossed by the left bronchus, and at the oesophageal hiatus.

The stomach is simple, similar to that of the dog or cat, and varies considerably in size and position depending on its fullness. It sits in the cranial abdomen and fits into the caudal curve of the liver. The pylorus can be distinguished readily. The small intestine consists of duodenum, ileum and jejunum, and is approximately 1.9 m in length and 5 mm in diameter, although the separate regions are not easily distinguishable grossly. There is no caecum or ileocolic valve, the small and large intestines merging in the caudal abdomen adjacent to the mesenteric lymph node. The colon is short, the combined lengths of the ascending, transverse and descending parts being only about 10 cm.

The liver is relatively large, and has six lobes: left lateral, left medial, quadrate, right medial, right lateral and caudate. The gall bladder is pear shaped and lies between the quadrate and right medial lobes. The bile duct enters the proximal duodenum with the pancreatic duct. The pancreas is V-shaped, and pink or red in colour. It has two parts, one extending down the descending duodenum and the other occupying the area between stomach and spleen. The spleen itself is crescent shaped and grey-brown in colour, and measures $5 \times 2 \times 0.8$ cm approximately.

Respiratory system

The respiratory system consists of the nasal passages, the pharynx, the larynx, the trachea, and the lungs. The nasal cavity is separated by the nasal septum into right and left portions, both of which join the pharynx at the nasopharyngeal opening. The Eustachian tubes open into the nasopharynx via slit-like openings on the wall of the cavity, joining the middle ear with the pharynx. The larynx consists of thyroid, cricoid, and arytenoid cartilages and the epiglottis. The trachea is approximately 9 cm long, and extends from the larynx to the tracheal bifurcation in the mid-thorax, at the level of the fifth intercostal space. It is made from 60–70 C-shaped cartilage rings.

The lungs occupy the cone shaped thoracic cavity from the first to the tenth intercostal spaces. The caudal surface of each lung is concave, and is in contact with the dome shaped diaphragm. The diaphragm itself has a sternal part, attached to the xiphoid cartilage and the cartilage of the last five ribs, costal parts which are attached to the ribs, and a dorsal part which attaches by two tendinous 'legs' or crura to the dorsal wall. These crura may extend caudally as far as the last lumbar vertebra The left lung has apical and diaphragmatic lobes, separated by an oblique fissure at the level of the sixth or seventh intercostal space. The heart lies adjacent to the caudal part of the apical lobe. The right lung has apical, middle, diaphragmatic and accessory lobes, with the apical and middle lobes forming a cardiac notch.

The heart and arteries

The heart extends approximately from the sixth to eighth rib. It is cone shaped, and lies with the apex to the left of the midline. The ligament which joins the heart to the sternum is often associated with the deposition of quantities of fat, and on lateral radiography the heart shadow appears to be raised above the sternum. Loss of this space can be an indicator of cardiac enlargement. The aortic arch gives rise to the brachiocephalic trunk, then the left subclavian artery before turning caudally. The brachiocephalic trunk splits into left and right common carotid arteries and right subclavian artery at the level of the thoracic inlet.

Urogenital system

The kidneys are retroperitoneal, and are situated in the sublumbar region either side of the spinal column, aorta and vena cava. The right kidney is most cranial, being embedded in a fossa of the caudate lobe of the liver. The cranial pole of this kidney lies level with T14, with the right adrenal gland just cranial to it. The left

kidney lies with its cranial pole just caudal to the first lumbar vertebra. The ureters run along the ventral surface of the sublumbar
muscles and enter the dorsolateral surface of the bladder just caudal
to the bladder neck. The bladder itself sits just cranial to the pelvic
inlet and measures approximately 2 cm in length by 1 cm diameter
when empty. The urethra originates from the bladder at the level of
the pelvic inlet. In the female, it extends caudally and opens into the
ventral floor of the vagina in the vaginovestibular junction. In the
male, an area of prostatic tissue surrounds the base of the bladder,
and the urethra passes through it. It extends caudally to exit the
pelvic canal, then loops cranioventrally, ventral to the os penis, to
the preputial opening in the midventral abdomen, caudal to the
umbilicus. The prepuce consists of a fold of skin which is hairy on
the exterior, but glabrous (hairless) within the fold.

The female genital tract consists of paired ovaries, situated caudal
to the kidneys. The uterus consists of fallopian tubes and long,
tapering uterine horns which fuse into a short body. The vagina is
short, 1.5–1.8 cm long, and exits in the vulva. In the immature and
anoestrous ferret, the labial folds are soft and small. When in oestrus, the folds become enlarged and swollen (Figure 1.2 (a) and (b)).

The male genital tract consists of paired scrotal sacs situated
beneath the anus, and the penis, composed of two corpora caver-
nosa originating from the ischial tuberosities which fuse as they turn
cranially to form the body of the penis. From the testis and epidi-
dymis, the vas deferens passes cranially through the inguinal canal
on each side, loops over the ureter and through the prostate to join
the urethra. The urethra lies within the body of the penis surrounded
by the corpus spongiosum, which expands at the base and at the
distal end to form the bulb and glans of the penis respectively: the os
penis lies within the glans.

Nervous system

The brain of the ferret is simpler than that of other carnivores. The
forebrain is relatively narrow in the adult animal, reflecting the shape
of the skull, giving the forebrain a triangular appearance. Otherwise

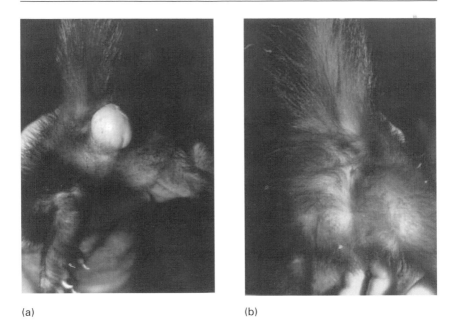

(a)   (b)

Figure 1.2 External genitalia of a female ferret, (a) in oestrus, compared with (b) anoestrus or immature animals.

the central and peripheral nervous systems resemble those seen in the dog and cat.

Skin and hair coat

The skin of ferrets is very thick, varying from 0.5 to 1.8 mm. It is particularly thick over the neck and shoulders. In the healthy animal, the skin should be smooth and free from scales. There are numerous sebaceous glands, and the sebaceous secretion spreads over the body to give the ferret a characteristic musky odour. The quantity of sebaceous secretion increases during the breeding season, producing an increase in odour, yellowing of the fur in albino animals, and an oily feel to the coat. There are no sweat glands in the skin: these are found only in the footpads and nose. They have paired anal glands situated either side of the anus, which produce a serous yellow liquid with a pungent odour, used to mark their territory. This secretion may be expressed by young or frightened animals, but cannot be projected over long distances and leads to only a momentary foul smell, contributing only a little to the overall odour of the animal. Older animals tend not to express their anal gland secretion so frequently.

The hair coat consists of long guard hairs, and a short soft undercoat. Ferrets moult in spring and autumn, and there are marked changes in the coat between the seasons which are controlled by the light:dark ratio, the hair being typically longer and softer with a thicker undercoat in the winter. Several colour variations are recognised in ferrets, particularly in the USA where there are more than thirty different varieties (see Plates 1 and 2). For example the typical polecat or fitch ferret has black guard hairs with a cream undercoat and a black mask and points, albino ferrets have white hair, and cinnamon or sandy ferrets have beige guard hairs with a cream undercoat and no mask. The mask configuration and overall colour may vary in individual animals from season to season, making identification of individuals in a colony by their appearance alone more difficult.

Reference

An, N.Q. and Evans, H.E. (1998) Anatomy of the ferret. In J.G. Fox (Ed) *Biology and Diseases of the Ferret*. 2nd edn. Williams and Wilkins, Baltimore, pp. 19–70.

2 BIOLOGY AND BEHAVIOUR

Biology

Ferrets generally live between five and nine years. Males (hobs) can be twice as large as females (jills), even if neutered. Both sexes exhibit seasonal fluctuations of up to 30–40% in body weight, as subcutaneous fat is added in the autumn and shed in the spring. They lack sweat glands in the skin and regulate their body temperature by panting and behavioural mechanisms, which renders them susceptible to overheating, particularly in humid conditions.

Cardiovascular system

The heart rate and blood pressure in the ferret are influenced by the animal's behaviour during measurement. The heart rate in anaesthetised ferrets has been measured at between 200 and 400 beats per minute, depending on the type of anaesthetic used. It is thought that there is little vagal tone, and there may be a high tonic sympathetic discharge leading to the relatively high heart rate. Systolic blood pressure is approximately 141–164 mmHg, and diastolic pressure 110–125 mmHg.

The pulmonary vasculature is very sensitive to hypoxia induced vasoconstriction, which is thought to be an adaptation to burrowing.

Ferrets generally have a higher packed cell volume than other domestic species, with a higher red cell count and high haemoglobin content.

Respiratory tract

The breathing rate in the conscious ferret is approximately 33 to 36 breaths per minute, with a tidal volume of approximately 6 ml. The ferret lung is large in relation to its body weight, and in conjunction with the flexibility of the thoracic wall, this is believed to be an adaptation to subterranean hunting. There are few epithelial nerves in the trachea, and the cough reflex is elicited by stimulation of the larynx, but not by stimulation of the trachea. The trachea is lined by ciliated epithelium, with numerous fluid secreting submucosal glands and some goblet cells, which increase in number towards the bronchi. Under normal conditions, very small amounts of fluid secretions are produced in the trachea, but fluid and mucus secretion may increase during stress or inhalation of irritants.

Gastro-intestinal tract

The ferret has five pairs of major salivary glands which produce different types of secretion when stimulated, the combined product being saliva which is hypotonic to plasma. Since ferrets tend to eat their food quickly, saliva probably plays little role in digestion, but may be important in lubricating food. The oesophagus consists entirely of striated muscle, the cervical and thoracic parts being lined by keratinised stratified squamous epithelium.

The stomach has a large capacity, adult ferrets may drink 100 ml of milk in a few minutes, but ferrets vomit readily in response to overstretching of the stomach or chemical stimulation. Retching or vomiting are often preceded by backwards movement, excess salivation, holding the head down and squinting. Under normal conditions, the majority of the food is stored in the stomach after eating, where it mixes with digestive enzymes and hydrochloric acid before passing into the small intestine. Both small and large intestine are short, leading to a short gut transit time: food passes through the entire intestine in only about three to four hours, so in order for the animal to be able to digest and absorb sufficient nutrients in this short time they must be given a highly digestible energy dense diet.

Urinary system

Morphologically, the kidneys are similar to other species. Urine production varies with the nature and composition of the diet, varying from 8 to 140 ml per day. Ferrets have a marked ability to concentrate their urine, samples sometimes reaching 2000 mOsm/l, and this may indicate the origin of the ferret as a desert dwelling animal. High levels of protein may also be found in urine from normal animals. Males frequently have very dark coloured urine, which can give false positive results for ketonuria when using test strips, since the urine is a similar colour to the strip.

Special senses

Ferrets have relatively poor vision, although they are able to spot moving objects at close range reasonably well, and they may be able to distinguish some colours. They rely more on hearing and smell. They have an extensive turbinate system and probably have a keen sense of smell. Their auditory system is relatively poorly developed at birth, but becomes fully functional by 42 days, after which time they have sensitive hearing and are able to localise sounds well. They respond best to frequencies of sound in the range 4–15 kHz, but lactating females appear able to hear the high frequency cries of neonatal animals and will turn towards them, these sounds being above 16 kHz.

Behaviour

Ferrets are closely related to the European polecat (*Mustela putorius*), and can interbreed with them, but are less temperamental and more docile while retaining many of their natural and instinctive behaviour patterns. Ferrets are lively, playful and curious, do not develop a fear of humans or human environments, and will be tractable and friendly if handled when young, although jills become very aggressive and protective of their young when nursing. They will readily enter narrow, dark tunnels resembling the burrows of rabbits and other prey animals, and will benefit from plastic tubes, cardboard boxes and climbing frames placed within their environments to simulate the natural situation (see Plate 3). Young ferrets like to chew their playthings, so care must be taken when choosing these items that they will not be swallowed leading to gastrointestinal obstructions. Latex rubber items should be avoided in particular.

Ferrets spend up to 75% of their time asleep, and like to sleep in dark, enclosed areas, so wooden or cardboard nest boxes should be provided: ferrets will even sleep in groups in large paper bags. In the remainder of the time, they will play intensively and explore new environments enthusiastically, spending much time burrowing through their bedding causing them to sneeze, which is quite normal provided sneezing is not overly frequent or associated with a nasal discharge or other clinical signs. Exercise periods often coincide with feeding times, and may be followed by rest periods.

Ferrets are naturally gregarious, and can be kept in compatible pairs or groups without aggression, particularly if there is ample environmental enrichment. Aggressive encounters usually involve copious screaming as one animal bites another on the neck or shoulder: the thick skin in this region usually prevents serious injury, and it is normal for males to grasp females in this area during mating.

Ferrets are able to vocalise and produce a number of different noises to accompany their activities. When playing, they may hiss and chuckle, when fighting, frightened or threatened, they may emit a loud screaming noise, and when foraging they may produce a low pitched grumble.

Young ferrets will play constantly. Mock aggression, play chasing, pouncing and wrestling are common activities. They will nip playfully at anything, trying out their teeth, and will bite when first handled. They will become more friendly if handled frequently, and if play biting persists it can be discouraged by pushing the knuckles into the animal's mouth a few times.

3 MANAGEMENT AND NUTRITION

Ferrets are adaptable creatures and will readily take to life as a pet. They can be kept successfully in a variety of conditions, indoors and outdoors, ranging from animals held in cages like rabbits or guinea pigs to 'free range' ferrets which have the run of the owner's house. Females and young males benefit from being kept in groups, but breeding and pregnant jills and mature males may need to be kept singly to reduce aggression and maximise fertility.

Housing

Given the choice, a ferret will build itself a burrow incorporating a sleeping area, larder for storage of food, several escape holes and a separate latrine area, usually a vertical surface against which the animal will defaecate. Housing should provide as natural an environment as possible in order to ensure the physical and psychological well being of the animals. If the environment is suitable, animals can be kept outdoors or indoors. An artificial warren can easily be created using plastic tubes, small branches, cardboard boxes and paper bags, providing a sleeping area or nest box where the animal can remain hidden from view, a larder area, and a vertical surface to act as a latrine area which can be cleaned out as necessary. A well designed natural enclosure such as this will provide the animals with ample environmental enrichment, allowing the animals to exhibit natural behaviour and reducing aggressive encounters.

Ferrets are sociable creatures and should be kept in compatible pairs or groups wherever possible. Jills (without litters), young animals before puberty and castrated males (hobbles) are suitable for being group housed, and a jill and a hob may be kept together, although they may fight when a litter is born and are best separated for this period. In general, it is better to keep the animals in pairs or groups in large pens with room for exercise and plenty of playthings, rather than to allow them to roam free in the house all the time (see Plate 4). Cages and pens can be bought commercially or may be constructed from welded wire mesh attached to a wooden frame. They should have solid floors and be lined with a thick layer of bedding to absorb any urine or faeces, and to give the animals a substrate to burrow and play in. Glass tanks are unsuitable because the ventilation within them is poor. A nest box placed within the pen made from cardboard or wood, lined with bedding material such as paper wool, wood shavings, good quality straw or artificial sheep-skin, will provide security and a sleeping area.

Young animals in particular have a tendency to gnaw objects in the environment, and will burrow into furniture etc. wherever possible. This may result in destruction of the environment and can predispose to dental damage or gastro-intestinal obstructions. In addition, they are good escape artists and will squeeze through even tiny gaps, so accommodation must be designed with care and rendered 'ferret-proof', with secure fastenings.

Ferrets kept in smaller cages should be allowed out for exercise regularly.

Ferrets are clean animals and will usually use one corner of the cage or pen as a latrine, leaving the rest of the pen clean. This area can be cleaned out once or twice daily, the bedding in the rest of the pen being changed once or twice weekly. The whole cage or pen should be disinfected weekly. Ferrets can be house trained and will learn to use litter boxes, but the short gut transit time means they may not always be able to reach litter boxes in time if they are far away, so free range ferrets need to have several litter boxes sited in convenient places throughout the home.

Ferrets thrive in temperatures between 15 and 24°C, but will adapt to colder temperatures (7–10°C) reasonably well. Unweaned kits should be kept at a higher temperature (15°C). However, they have difficulty tolerating temperatures above 30°C, particularly if combined with high humidity. The optimum humidity is between 40 and 65%. If they are to be kept outdoors or in an uncontrolled environment, shelters should be provided to protect the animals from draughts and extremes of temperature. It is important for all ferrets that there is adequate ventilation, to reduce the odour and because they are susceptible to respiratory diseases.

Nutrition

Ferrets are efficient hunters and their natural diet consists mainly of a mixture of small mammals, with some birds, fish, amphibia and invertebrates. These are eaten whole, providing valuable vitamins and minerals as well as protein, and are usually eaten fresh, although sometimes carcasses will be stored for consumption later.

Little research has been done on the exact nutritional needs of ferrets, and much has been extrapolated from the dietary needs of mink and other carnivores. The following contains information taken from several authors who have reared ferrets successfully.

When formulating diets for ferrets, important considerations are the energy concentration of the diet, the amino acid composition of dietary protein, and the digestibility of the protein. Ferrets are strict carnivores and require a diet high in protein and fat but low in fibre. There seems to be little absolute requirement for carbohydrate provided there is sufficient protein and fat in the diet to provide substrates for gluconeogenesis. Their capacity to digest complex carbohydrates is low, although disaccharides are digested efficiently. They eat to calorie requirements, and the high metabolic rate and short gut transit time mean they need highly digestible diets with a high energy density and protein level. Diets rich in carbohydrates may lead to protein and fat deficiencies. Under natural conditions, they will eat up to nine or ten small meals daily, although twice daily feeding is acceptable. Ensure any old food is removed.

Adult ferrets need approximately 840–1260 kJ/kg (200–300 kcal/kg) body weight daily. High energy diets with up to 21 000 kJ/kg (5000 kcal/kg) diet may be needed for growth and reproduction.

Diets for adult ferrets should contain 30–40% protein, and breeding and young animals should have a minimum protein level of 35%. Fat enhances the palatability and texture of the diet, and delays gastric emptying leading to a feeling of satiety. However, the fat content needs to be restricted or protein and mineral intake may be insufficient. A level of 18–20% fat is sufficient, and up to 15% of the fat should be in the form of unsaturates, containing essential fatty acids such as linoleic acid. Unsaturated fatty acids have a tendency to become rancid, which results in unpalatability and destruction of vitamin E, so ferret diets should contain adequate levels of vitamin E (see Table 3.1) and be stored appropriately. Deficiencies in vitamin E predispose to steatitis (yellow fat disease).

Generally, ferrets fare well if given dry cat or kitten pellets with an appropriate protein level, which can be soaked and fed as a stiff paste, supplemented with pieces of meat or small amounts of moist cat food. Commercial ferret diets are also available. Canned cat food or dog food contain insufficient protein for ferrets, leading to subtle changes in the hair coat and poor reproductive efficiency, and may increase the incidence of dental calculus. Diets rich in plant derived proteins are associated with urolithiasis in mustelids. Ferrets like eggs and will appreciate these as an occasional treat. Often, natural ingredient diets are used, and these can be more palatable than commercial pellets, so although their nutritional value may be less, the animal eats more and therefore still satisfies its daily needs.

The vitamin and mineral requirements have not been determined precisely: Table 3.1 gives details of dietary levels which have been found to be suitable.

Fresh water should be provided ad lib in cups or bowls, and on average an adult ferret drinks 75–100 ml water daily. Ferrets play with their water so care should be taken to ensure that they have sufficient and that the bedding does not become too wet. Ferrets will also drink milk (see Plate 5), but excess should not be given as this predisposes to loose faeces. Water containers should not be galvanised, as this may lead to zinc toxicity.

Table 3.1   Nutritional requirements of ferrets.

Nutrient	Dietary content		Comments
Energy	kJ/kg	21 000	High energy density required
	(i.e. kcal/kg)	≤5000)	
Protein	%	30–40	Min 35 for growth or production
Fat	%	18–20	High unsaturate level required
Carbohydrate	%	22–44	No absolute requirement
Fibre	%	2–5	Low level required
Vitamins			
A	i.u./kg	33 600	1000–4200 i.u./kg body weight daily
D	i.u./kg	3667	65–325 i.u./kg body weight daily. May depend on Ca and P level and exposure to UV light
E	i.u./kg	125	3–15 i.u./kg body weight daily. Need at least 0.5 mg vitamin E per g unsaturated fat in diet
K	mg/kg	1	
B_1 (Thiamine)	mg/kg	8.4–97.8	
B_2 (Riboflavin)	mg/kg	1.5–3	
B_6 (Pyridoxine)	mg/kg	1	
B_{12} (Cyanocobalamin)	mg/kg	0.12	2–13 µg/kg body weight daily
Minerals			
Calcium	%	1.1–2.2	⎫ Need calcium:phosphorus ratio of at least 1.2, and an adequate vitamin D level
Phosphorus	%	0.9–1.2	⎬
Sodium chloride	%	≤1	
Magnesium	%	0.16–0.28	Depends also on Ca and P level
Zinc	mg/kg	105–215	Deficiency may lead to skin lesions in kits
Iodine	mg/kg	3–5	

Methods of identification

Microchip transponders provide a permanent method of identification which is free from side effects. The transponder should be implanted under the skin between the shoulder blades, and can be inserted using a hollow needle. The skin is tough in this area and it may be necessary to implant the device surgically under general anaesthesia through a stab incision, particularly in adult males. Close the incision with a single suture or with tissue adhesive.

Individual animals may be identified by their appearance, since the mask configuration varies between fitch (polecat) ferrets. However, this is not possible for albino animals, and seasonal changes in the pelage can make identification difficult in fitch animals as individuals vary year to year.

Animals may have their name or ID number permanently tattooed on the inside of the thigh. Shave the hair and sedate the animal for tattooing.

Collars can be used, however the thick neck and narrow head of the ferret make it easy for the animal to remove the collar so they have to be applied quite tightly. When placing collars on young animals, check very frequently that the collar is not restricting the animal's breathing or cutting into the skin.

Ear tags designed for use in small animals can be inserted on the lateral part of the pinna away from the central vessels. Ear tags are prone to being pulled out, particularly in group housed animals, leading to lacerations of the pinna, and in any case can be difficult to read due to their small size (see Plate 1).

Marker dyes applied to the coat can provide a temporary method for marking animals. This certainly is feasible in albino animals, but becomes more difficult with fitch (polecat) ferrets. Markers need to be reapplied frequently.

4 BREEDING

Ferrets become sexually mature in the spring following birth at approximately 8 to 12 months of age. They are seasonal breeders, females being active between March and September, and males from December to July. The breeding season is determined by photoperiod, responses being mediated via the pineal body, and can be manipulated by changes in the light cycle. Year round breeding can be achieved by keeping half the colony in a reverse lighting pattern, with summer light cycles in the winter and vice versa. It is important to keep ferrets in natural daylight or an appropriate artificial light cycle, since inappropriate photoperiods may cause problems. For example, kits reared on 12:12 light:dark cycles from birth may never come into breeding condition, and females kept continually in stimulatory photoperiods (14 hours light) will have three or four litters in succession, then eventually fail to conceive. A period of five to six weeks in winter cycles is then needed.

In both sexes, the hair coat is shed in the late spring, and in the autumn a thick undercoat develops which gives the coat a paler, rather fluffy appearance. Partial alopecia may be noted during the breeding season. In the male, hair loss begins from October to November under natural lighting conditions, and regrows at the end of the breeding season. In the female, hair loss may be noted following the first ovulation, and will recur after subsequent ovulations.

In the male, testicular development is stimulated by short day length. It begins in December and is completed by February or March, when the animal is ready to breed. Once maturity is reached, the testes are found in the subcutaneous tissue of the caudoventral abdomen, and they enlarge and descend into the scrotum only between December and July during the breeding season. Enlargement is due to development of the germinal epithelium and tubular lumen, and growth of the Sertoli and interstitial cells. Between August and December, when the animal is not breeding, the testes shrink. Their breeding season can be prolonged by keeping them permanently in a short photoperiod (six to eight hours light), when they may remain in breeding condition for more than one year, but a period of four to six weeks quiescence is then needed. Breeding efficiency declines after approximately three years of age.

Females are seasonally polyoestrous between March and September, the onset of oestrus being triggered by increasing day length. Jills are sensitive to the effects of extended daylight in the winter, and may be brought into heat out of season if exposed to artificial light. Long days (14 hours daylight) are needed for breeding to occur, although prolonged exposure to daylight can inhibit reproduction. Towards the end of the season, the reduced light intensity can lead to failure of implantation and poor breeding efficiency. The onset of sexual maturity can be advanced by keeping immature females in short days (six to eight hours) until beyond 90 days of age, then exposing to long days (over 14 hours). Oestrus will occur about four weeks after the change in lighting. This can bring them into breeding condition from four to five months of age.

Although females are seasonally polyoestrous, they are induced ovulators and will remain in heat for three to six months if not mated. Oestrus can be recognised by enlargement of the vulva (see Figure 1.2), which will reach maximum size one month after the onset of oestrus, and a mucoserous vaginal discharge. Behavioural changes which may be noted include increased irritability, decreased food intake, and reduced sleeping time. The high levels of oestrogen present during oestrus can be detrimental to the animal's health (see Chapter 9, Endocrine Diseases). Oestrous jills will lose weight and hair during the breeding season, and often develop a normocytic, normochromic anaemia, and after an initial leucocytosis and thrombocytosis, leucopenia and thrombocytopenia develop after about eight weeks. It is recommended that females which are not to be bred should be spayed at six to eight months of age. Following mating, the vulva will begin to dry up after three to four days, and will regress completely within four weeks, or longer towards the end of the breeding season or if oestrus was prolonged initially.

It is best to breed the animals early in the season, so the jill is not in oestrus for too long. In addition, high temperatures reduce fertility in the male and may affect implantation, parturition and lactation in the female, so mating early in the season results in maximum fecundity.

Mating

Females should be mated approximately 14 days after the vulval swelling appears, although conception can occur soon after the onset of vulval swelling. Mating will only occur when the female is ready: the male may try to mount her before this but will not succeed and may cause injury to the jill, so they should not be put together until the appropriate time. Take the female to the male, observe the pair for a few minutes after introduction, and separate them if fighting ensues. Mating can be vigorous, prolonged and noisy. The male will usually grasp the female by the scruff of the neck and drag her around the cage for up to one hour prior to coitus, which can then take a further one to three hours. This rough treatment seems to be essential to induce ovulation, which occurs 30–35 hours after mating. Male and female can be left together for a few days to allow repeat matings. Sperm can survive 36–48 hours in the female genital tract, and can penetrate ovarian follicles allowing for fertilisation prior to ovulation. The vulva dries up within a few days, and regresses between one and three weeks after copulation. The embryo implants in the uterine wall 12–13 days after fertilisation, and gestation lasts 40–44 days (average 42). The placenta is zonary and of the endotheliochorial type. Pregnancy can be confirmed by abdominal palpation from 14 days, when the fetuses will be the size of small walnuts, or by ultrasound from about 12 days, when the swollen uterine horns are visible.

If fertilisation does not occur, there will be a pseudopregnancy lasting 40–42 days, after which time there will be enlargement of the vulva signalling a return to oestrus. This will also occur 10–14 days after weaning or termination of the pregnancy provided there is sufficient light (16 hours daily), and the female may be mated again if she is in sufficiently good condition. Females which are mated first at the beginning of the season may therefore have two litters in one year. Jills will usually have three or four litters, but breeding performance declines after the third breeding season.

Pregnancy, parturition and lactation

Gestation lasts 40–44 days. Gestation length decreases with increasing day length and litter size, but increases with maternal age by approximately five hours with each pregnancy. Pregnant jills may be returned to their stable groups for the first half of pregnancy, but may become irritable and disturbed by their companions in the last two weeks, so can be separated to minimise the risk of cannibalism once the young are born. During gestation, the jill will lose her winter coat and may look rather scruffy, and it is important that she gets adequate nutrition. She needs to be fed ad lib a diet containing 35–40% protein, and 18–20% fat during pregnancy, increasing the fat content to 30% during lactation.

Nest boxes with a peephole entrance and suitable bedding material such as shredded paper, wood shavings or soft straw can be provided: jills may or may not choose to use these, some animals preferring to make nests outside the nest box or using their usual bedding material.

The jill needs to be observed during parturition because dystocia is fairly common, although it is best to disturb her as little as possible during birth, or she may delay parturition, continuing when the disturbance has passed, or cannibalise the young. This may also occur if there is any disturbance during the first few days after birth, or following fluctuations in environmental temperature. Inexperienced jills may ignore their kits altogether, choosing to mother toys or even humans instead. Parturition is usually very rapid, being completed within two to three hours. Between one and twelve kits weighing 6–12 g each are born: the average litter size is eight. They are born with their eyes and ears closed, and are covered with a fine hair coat which turns grey after three days in fitch animals, but remains white in albinos. They have a large fat pad at the back of the neck, with apocrine sweat glands in the skin which produce a secretion allowing the jill to recognise her kits. The eyes open from 28–34 days, the animals begin hearing from 32 days, and they become mobile and able to recognise the mother before their eyes open. During lactation, the jill becomes very sensitive to the high frequency sounds produced by neonatal kits. The young will stay in the nest box for the first two to three weeks, and the jill will retrieve them if they crawl out. Initially, she will lick the perineum of each kit to stimulate urination and defaecation, but this becomes spontaneous when the kits begin eating solid food prior to weaning.

Kits have voracious appetites, and the jill needs to produce copious amounts of milk. Kits will nurse immediately if they are warm and the jill curls around them, they will then attach to the nipples and stay there. Hungry kits can be recognised because they cry continually. Jills have eight nipples, but can feed more kits than this if the milk supply is good. Ferret milk contains 23.5% solids, composed of 34% fat, 25.5% protein, and 16.2% carbohydrate. If there are more than five kits, it is likely that return to oestrus will be suppressed by lactation. If not, the jill may return to oestrus before weaning. In this case, she should be mated again, since an excess of oestrogen can reduce the milk supply. Kits begin eating solid food from two to three weeks, and can be weaned at six to eight weeks, when they weigh at least 200–250 g. At this time they will eat about 30 g solid food daily and drink about 125 ml water.

Neonatal mortality can be high in ferrets, sometimes reaching 8–10%, due to stillbirths, congenital defects or cannibalism. Cannibalism is more common with larger litters, but can be an inherited trait. Kits may also die from hypothermia or bloat, which occurs if the kits overeat or if hygiene is poor. Good management will prevent these problems. Mortality reduces after five days – deaths after this time are usually due to maternal neglect or agalactia, which are more common if oestrus is induced prematurely. Leaving the mother undisturbed for several days post partum and ensuring she has adequate nutrition should reduce this problem. The jill should be given increasing quantities of food from two to three days after birth. Calcium supplementation may be needed to prevent hypocalcaemia (milk fever), which can occur at peak lactation three to four weeks after birth.

The transfer of antibodies to provide immunity for the young occurs through the passage of immunoglobulins across the intestinal mucosa. Gut closure occurs late in ferrets: transmucosal uptake of IgG can continue for the first 30 days of life, and IgG levels in the kits reach adult levels within two weeks. IgA and IgM are present but not concentrated in milk so levels in the kit remain low until active immunity begins (from about six weeks). Maternal immunity wanes from six to eight weeks.

The kits double their birth weight in the first five days, grow gradually up to four or five weeks, then grow rapidly to about 16 weeks when adult weight is reached. There is marked sexual dimorphism in body weight, males being twice as large as females, and this begins to become apparent from seven weeks (Figure 4.1).

Hand rearing

Kits may need to be hand reared or fostered, if there is a large litter, in cases of maternal agalactia, or if the mother dies. If the mother is still alive, she can provide warmth and protection and stimulate urination and defaecation. If she has died, then hand rearing involves providing these functions as well. Hand rearing is difficult, but can be successful provided an appropriate feeding schedule is adhered to. Canine or feline milk replacer can be used to feed them, although kits really need ferret milk for the first ten days and hand rearing from before this time is often unsuccessful. It is important to stick to a routine, feeding milk at body temperature at set times and ensuring strict hygiene. Initially, kits may need to be fed every two hours, using a small feeding bottle. Feed until the kit is satisfied, but do not overfeed as this predisposes to bloat. An appropriate volume can usually be found by trial and error. From two to three weeks,

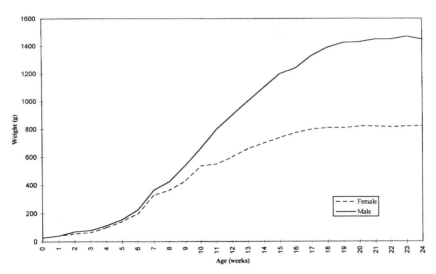

Figure 4.1   Growth of kits (adapted from Shump and Shump, 1978).

begin offering solid foods. Offer the kits some of the jill's food softened with water and with animal fat added (making a 30% fat content) to improve palatability. More details on hand rearing of ferret kits can be found in Chapter 11 and in Porter and Brown, (1997).

Orphaned kits may also be fostered onto other jills. The kits should be allowed to mix with the foster mother's own kits beforehand to acquire their smell in order to prevent rejection.

References

Porter, V. and Brown, N. (1997). *The Complete Book of Ferrets*. D & M Publications, Bedford.

Shump, A.V. and Shump, K.A. (1978) Growth and development of the European ferret (*Muskela putorius*). *Laboratory Animal Science*, **28**, p. 89.

5 ROUTINE PREVENTIVE CARE

Ferrets, like dogs and cats, will benefit from a suitable programme of preventive care, to reduce the incidence of husbandry related disorders and to allow for early detection of serious diseases. Preparation of a client handout giving details of recommended husbandry regimes and common disease problems can be very useful. The owner should check the animal's general condition as often as possible, looking for general signs of ill thrift, obesity or weight loss. The teeth should be checked for dental calculus or fractures, skin and hair coat for evidence of dermatitis, parasites or alopecia, ears for evidence of *Otodectes cynotis* which is common in ferrets, and anal area for evidence of diarrhoea. The nails may need trimming, depending on what environment the animal is kept in and whether they are able to wear the claws down burrowing in the environment.

The animal's housing should provide warmth and comfort, keeping the animals clean and dry. It should be designed to provide environmental enrichment, giving the animals sufficient room and a variety of suitable playthings to allow them to satisfy their natural curiosity. However, they will chew readily at anything soft, so care must be taken that they are not exposed to small or easily destructible items which could be swallowed causing an intestinal foreign body.

Ferrets have a musky odour which tends to be stronger during the breeding season, due to an increase in sebaceous secretions. Bathing the animal in mild shampoo may reduce the odour temporarily, but should not be carried out more than once or twice monthly or it may cause drying of the skin.

Young ferrets should be brought for a health check and first vaccination some time after six to eight weeks of age, and then brought for an annual check up until 4–5 years old. This may include faecal screening for pathogens such as *Salmonella* and *Campylobacter*, and blood sampling for haematology, serology, and biochemistry. Older animals are more prone to metabolic, endocrine, cardiovascular, urogenital and neoplastic diseases, and benefit from twice yearly health checks. Table 5.1 gives an example of a health monitoring protocol for ferrets.

Table 5.1 Routine health monitoring schedule for pet ferrets.

6 or 8*	1st distemper vaccine if needed (endemic areas), faecal screen
10–12*	2nd distemper vaccine if needed
12–14	1st (or 3rd) distemper vaccine, rabies vaccine if required, faecal screen
26–32	Spay or castrate, faecal screen
1 year	Rabies booster if required (annual)
3 years	Distemper booster (every 1–3 years)

* Earlier vaccination for kits of non-vaccinated dams
Routine health checks are recommended annually until four to five years of age, then every six months. Animals of unknown origin should be tested for Aleutian disease virus.

Ferrets should be vaccinated against canine distemper, preferably using a monovalent modified live distemper vaccine of non-ferret cell origin. If only polyvalent vaccines are available, the canine parvovirus fraction should be killed. Choose a vaccine in which the distemper fraction has been made from the Onderstepoort strain grown in the Vero cell line (derived from the green monkey). Other strains may be insufficiently attenuated and cause disease. No vaccines are currently licensed for use in ferrets in the UK. At the time of going to press, Nobivac DH℠ (Intervet) appears to be safe for ferrets and mink, however vaccine production changes continually and it is wise to check with the manufacturer. Half the recommended dog dose will provide immunity in ferrets. Where distemper is endemic, the first dose should be given at six weeks in kits of non-vaccinated dams or eight weeks in kits from vaccinated dams, to allow for waning of maternal immunity. Second and third doses should be given at 10–12 weeks and 13–14 weeks. Where distemper is not endemic, a single primary dose at 12 weeks is sufficient. Boosters are needed every one to three years. Adverse reactions are rare, but there may be vomiting and diarrhoea, erythema or pyrexia. If anaphylaxis occurs, give supportive treatment including adrenaline, antihistamines and fluids.

Ferrets are not regarded as susceptible to feline panleucopenia, canine parvovirus, leptospirosis or mink enteritis.

Imported animals currently need to enter quarantine on arrival in the UK and may need to be vaccinated against rabies, although this may change since quarantine requirements for dogs and cats are under review. Use killed vaccines such as Rabisin™ (Merial) as there have been cases of disease possibly related to the use of live rabies vaccine. Give the first dose at three to four months, with annual boosters. The supply and use of rabies vaccine has to be authorised by the MAFF. No rabies vaccines are licensed for use on ferrets and this should be discussed with the owner prior to administration. Ferrets of unknown health status should be tested on acquisition for Aleutian disease virus (see Chapter 8). This can be done using a sample of plasma collected by clipping a toenail and drawing the blood into a heparinised capillary tube. The plasma can be tested for the virus using counter-immuno-electrophoresis. Positive animals should not enter a colony since they present a health risk for the other animals, even if overtly well.

Some routine surgical procedures may need to be performed. Castrating males at six to eight months of age will reduce aggressive behaviour and odour. Females which are not to be bred should be spayed to prevent hyperoestrogenism due to persistent oestrus, which can result in an often fatal bone marrow depression.

Further reading

Chapter 1

An, N.Q. and Evans, H.E. (1998) Anatomy of the ferret. In J.G. Fox (ed.) *Biology and Diseases of the Ferret*. 2nd edn. Williams and Wilkins, Baltimore. pp. 19–70.

Andrews, P.L.R., Illman, O. and Mellersh, A. (1979) Some observations of anatomical abnormalities and disease states in a population of 350 ferrets (*Mustela furo L.*). *Zeitschrift für Versuchtierkunde*, **21**, pp. 346–53.

Brown, S.A. (1997) Basic anatomy, physiology and husbandry. In: E.V. Hillyer and K.E. Quesenberry (eds). *Ferrets, Rabbits and Rodents: Clinical Medicine and Surgery*. W.B. Saunders Company, Philadelphia, pp. 3–13.

Cooper, J.E. (1990) Skin diseases of ferrets. *The Veterinary Annual*, **30**, pp. 325–34.

Moody, K.D., Bowman, T.A. and Lang, C.M. (1985) Laboratory management of the ferret for biomedical research. *Laboratory Animal Science*, **35**(3), pp. 272–9.

Porter, V. and Brown, N. (1997) *The Complete Book of Ferrets*. D & M Publications, Bedford.

Chapter 2

Bernard, S.L., Gorham, J.R. and Ryland, R.M. (1984) Biology and diseases of ferrets: II-Biology. In: J.G. Fox, B.J. Cohen and F.M. Loew (eds). *Laboratory Animal Medicine*. Academic Press, Orlando. pp. 386–89.

Besch-Williford, C.L. (1987) Biology and medicine of the ferret. *Veterinary Clinics of North America: Small Animal Practice*, **17**, pp. 1155–83.

Brown, S.A. (1997) Basic anatomy, physiology and husbandry. In: E.V. Hillyer and K.E. Quesenberry (eds). *Ferrets, Rabbits and Rodents: Clinical Medicine and Surgery*. W.B. Saunders Company, Philadelphia, pp. 3–13.

Burke, T.J. (1988) Common diseases and medical management of ferrets. In: E.R. Jacobson and G.V. Kollias (eds). *Exotic Animals*. Churchill Livingstone, Edinburgh, pp. 247–60.

Moody, K.D., Bowman, T.A. and Lang, C.M. (1985) Laboratory management of the ferret for biomedical research. *Laboratory Animal Science*, **35**(3), pp. 272–9.

Porter, V. and Brown, N. (1997) *The Complete Book of Ferrets*. D & M Publications, Bedford.

Rosenthal, K. (1994) Ferrets. *Veterinary Clinics of North America*, **24**(1), pp. 1–23.

Ryland, L.M., Bernard, S.L. and Gorham, J.R. (1983) A clinical guide to the pet ferret. *Compendium of Continuing Education for the Practising Veterinarian*, **5**(1), pp. 25–32.

Whary, M.T. and Andrews, P.L.R. (1998) The physiology of the ferret. In: J.G. Fox, *Biology and Diseases of the Ferret*. 2nd edn. Williams and Wilkins, Baltimore, pp. 103–48.

Chapter 3

Besch-Williford, C.L. (1987) Biology and medicine of the ferret. *Veterinary Clinics of North America: Small Animal Practice*, **17**, pp. 1155–83.

Brown, S.A. (1997) Basic anatomy, physiology and husbandry. In: E.V. Hillyer and K.E. Quesenberry (eds). *Ferrets, Rabbits and Rodents: Clinical Medicine and Surgery*. W.B. Saunders Company, Philadelphia, pp. 3–13.

Fox, J.G. (1998) Housing and management. In: J.G. Fox (ed.) *Biology and Diseases of the Ferret*. 2nd edn. Williams and Wilkins, Baltimore, pp. 173–82.

Fox, J.G. and McLain, D.E. (1998) Nutrition. In: J.G. Fox (ed.) *Biology and Diseases of the Ferret*. 2nd edn. Williams and Wilkins, Baltimore, pp. 149–72.

Porter, V. and Brown, N. (1997) *The Complete Book of Ferrets*. D & M Publications, Bedford.

Wolfensohn, S.E. and Lloyd, M.H. (1998) *A Handbook of Laboratory Animal Management and Welfare*. Blackwell Science, Oxford.

Chapter 4

Besch-Williford, C.L. (1987) Biology and medicine of the ferret. *Veterinary Clinics of North America: Small Animal Practice*, **17**, pp. 1155–83.

Burke, T.J. (1988) Common diseases and medical management of ferrets.

In: E.R. Jacobson and G.V. Kollias (eds.). *Exotic Animals*. Churchill Livingstone, Edinburgh. pp. 247–60.

Fox, J.G. and Bell, J.A. (1998) Growth, reproduction and breeding. In: J.G. Fox (ed.). *Biology and Diseases of the Ferret*. 2nd edn. Williams and Wilkins, Baltimore, pp. 211–30.

Moody, K.D., Bowman, T.A. and Lang, C.M. (1985) Laboratory management of the ferret for biomedical research. *Laboratory Animal Science*, **35**(3), pp. 272–9.

Ryland, L.M. and Gorham, J.R. (1978) The ferret and its diseases. *Journal of the American Veterinary Medical Association*, **173**(9), pp. 1154–8.

Shump, A.U. and Shump, K.A. (1978) Growth and development of the European ferret (*Mustela putorius*). *Laboratory Animal Science*, **28**, p. 89.

Chapter 5

Besch-Williford, C.L. (1987) Biology and medicine of the ferret. *Veterinary Clinics of North America: Small Animal Practice*, **17**, pp. 1155–83.

Burke, T.J. (1988) Common diseases and medical management of ferrets. In: E.R. Jacobson and G.V. Kollias (eds). *Exotic Animals*. Churchill Livingstone, Edinburgh, pp. 247–60.

Marini, R.P. and Fox, J.G. (1998) Anaesthesia, surgery and biomethodology. In: J.G. Fox (ed.). *Biology and Diseases of the Ferret*. 2nd edn., Williams and Wilkins, Baltimore, pp. 449–84.

Oxenham, M. (1990) Distemper vaccination in ferrets (letter). *Veterinary Record*, **126**, p. 67.

Porter, V. and Brown, N. (1997) *The Complete Book of Ferrets*. D & M Publications, Bedford.

Quesenberry, K.E. (1997) Basic approach to veterinary care. In: E.V. Hillyer and K.E. Quesenberry (eds). *Ferrets, Rabbits and Rodents: Clinical Medicine and Surgery*. W.B. Saunders, Philadelphia, pp. 14–25.

Rosenthal, K. (1994) Ferrets. *Veterinary Clinics of North America: Small Animal Practice*, **24**, pp. 1–23.

Ryland, L.M. and Bernard, S.L. (1983) A clinical guide to the pet ferret. *Compendium on Continuing Education for the Practising Veterinarian*, **5**, pp. 25–32.

SECTION 2
DISEASES: A SYSTEMATIC APPROACH

6 DISEASES WITH RESPIRATORY SIGNS

Respiratory disease in ferrets can be due to a range of infectious and non-infectious causes as in other species. To differentiate the various causes, a well taken history, thorough clinical examination and radiography are essential, particularly for lower respiratory disease.

Canine distemper virus

Ferrets are prone to canine distemper virus, which produces an acute disease with nearly 100% mortality.

Aetiology and pathogenesis

CDV is a morbillivirus (family Paramyxoviridae), which is pantropic and replicates in all epithelioid and lymphoid organs. Only one antigenic strain is recognised, although different strains do vary in virulence, some strains having mainly respiratory signs whereas others have predominantly neurotropic signs. CDV causes profound suppression of cell mediated immunity, predisposing to secondary bacterial infection which complicates the clinical picture and may affect the outcome. The virus survives fairly well in the environment, and spreads efficiently by airborne droplets, animals becoming infected within hours of exposure to an infected animal. In addition, the virus is shed in nasal and ocular discharges, urine, faeces and skin scurf. Shedding of virus begins seven days after exposure. Dogs are the main source of distemper. Since the incidence of disease in dogs is very low in most parts of the UK, the disease is correspondingly rare in ferrets.

Clinical signs

Following exposure, there is a seven to nine day incubation period, then the animal develops a biphasic pyrexia, loses its appetite, and develops an initially serous then mucopurulent ocular and nasal discharge, which causes the eyelids to stick together. There may be photophobia and blepharospasm. On day 10–12 a rash develops under the chin and in the inguinal area (this may be the first thing noticed by the owner), and there may be keratitis of the footpads producing classical hardpad. The disease progresses to tracheitis, bronchitis and severe bronchopneumonia. Death usually follows on day 12–14 for ferret adapted strains, and day 21–25 for canine adapted strains. If animals survive this catarrhal phase, they will develop a CNS phase within a few weeks, characterised by hyperexcitability, excess salivation, muscle tremor, convulsion, coma and death. Vomiting and diarrhoea are uncommon in ferrets with canine distemper virus.

Diagnosis

The signs are typical, and CDV should be suspected in unvaccinated ferrets of any age showing these signs. The diagnosis can be confirmed by virus isolation; alternatively immunofluorescence can be performed on smears of conjunctival epithelium or blood from the live animal, or lymph node, bladder epithelium or cerebellum from post mortem specimens. Typical distemper inclusion bodies may be demonstrated in conjunctival epithelium, urinary bladder or tracheal epithelium. Fluorescent antibody tests may be positive before the onset of clinical signs, aiding a rapid diagnosis. Recently, reverse transcriptase polymerase chain reaction (RT-PCR) has been used to detect active virus in mononuclear cells in experimentally infected ferrets, and this may become a useful diagnostic test in future.

Treatment and control

No treatment is indicated, and affected animals should be euthanased. Prophylactic vaccination is recommended (see Chapter 5). In
the face of an outbreak, separate affected animals as soon as possible to reduce spread, and vaccinate healthy animals immediately.
Immune serum (Maxagloban P℠, Hoechst) can be used to provide
passive immunity: give 0.2 ml by subcutaneous or intramuscular
injection to provide passive immunity for two to three weeks, but do
not give it at the same time as a vaccination.

Influenza

Several strains of mammalian (particularly human) influenza virus
are capable of infecting ferrets. The disease in adult ferrets is usually
mild, but it can prove fatal in kits.

Aetiology and pathogenesis

Influenza virus is an orthomyxovirus capable of rapid antigenic
variation. Ferrets usually catch it from personnel incubating the
infection, and it can then spread by droplets from ferret to ferret, or
back to people. The virus replicates in the upper respiratory tract,
causing catarrhal inflammation leading to congestion, oedema and
some necrosis in the nasal mucosa.

Clinical signs

Clinical signs may develop as soon as 48 hours after exposure.
Affected animals develop a biphasic fever (40–41°C), they become
anorexic and listless, then begin sneezing and coughing, with a nasal
discharge. There may be sensitivity to light. The disease rarely
progresses beyond this stage, and recovery usually follows rapidly
after the second pyrexic episode, within 7–14 days of first exposure.
Recovery is followed by a short period of immunity to reinfection by
the same strain of virus. Occasionally, the disease may progress to

pneumonia. Neonates may have a more severe form and are more likely to die from lower respiratory infections.

Diagnosis

Initially, the respiratory signs are similar to those of canine distemper, but the disease is mild and recovery begins after a few days. Diagnosis can be confirmed by virus isolation or rising antibody titres. Other causes of pneumonia (bacterial and fungal) can be ruled out on the basis of duration and response to treatment.

Treatment and control

No treatment is required, and recovery begins spontaneously within a few days. Occasionally, antibiotics may be required to control secondary infection. Supportive therapy including palatable foods and fluids can be given at home. Vaccination is not indicated, since protection is short lived and there are many antigenically distinct strains of the virus.

Pneumonia

Aetiology and pathogenesis

Occasionally, bacteria such as *Streptococcus zooepidemicus* or *Pasteurella pneumotropica* may invade the respiratory tract as primary pathogens, but it is more common for bacterial pneumonia to develop secondarily to viral infections or other diseases. Organisms such as *E. coli*, *Proteus vulgaris*, *Klebsiella pneumoniae* and *Pseudomonas aeruginosa* can cause pneumonia secondary to diseases such as influenza virus infection, Aleutian disease, cardiomyopathy, immunosuppression or lymphoid neoplasia with synergistic effects. Aspiration pneumonia can occur as a sequela to orally administered medicines or vomitus. Mycobacteriosis may occur but is most common in the mesenteric lymph nodes.

Clinical signs

There may be any or all of the following signs: nasal discharge, dyspnoea, an increase in abdominal respiration, lethargy, anorexia and cyanosis. There may also be fever depending on the cause. Occasionally, there may be a fulminant pneumonia with sepsis which causes acute death with few clinical signs.

Diagnosis

The history and clinical signs are indicative of lower respiratory infection. Radiography will reveal increased density in the lung fields, with air bronchograms, hilar oedema, or other typical features depending on the cause of the pneumonia. A definitive diagnosis may be made by culture of tracheal exudates or examination of post mortem specimens. There may be consolidation of the cranioventral lung lobes, and with aspiration pneumonia necrosis of the airways and surrounding alveoli may be present. There may be a granulomatous response in chronic cases.

Treatment and control

Treatment with oxygen or diuretics may improve the animal's gas exchange, and fluids and force feeding may improve the animal's general condition. Give antibiotic therapy according to sensitivities in cases of bacterial pneumonia. Penicillins, potentiated sulphonamides or enrofloxacin may all be effective. Further cases can be prevented depending on the cause by taking care with oral administration of medicines, isolating affected animals, and dealing with any predisposing factors appropriately.

Other diseases with respiratory signs

Conditions such as pulmonary mycosis, primary or secondary neoplasia, or malignant hyperthermia may present with apparently respiratory signs. Pleural effusion may occur secondarily to neoplasms in the thoracic cavity, and lead to respiratory signs.

Cardiomyopathy

This can lead to respiratory signs due to pulmonary congestion and oedema and pleural effusion. This condition is discussed in Chapter 12, Cardiovascular Diseases.

Trauma

Ferrets which fall from a height or are involved in road traffic accidents may present with pneumothorax or rupture of the diaphragm as in dogs and cats, and may be treated as these species.

Endogenous lipid pneumonia

Multiple coalescing white or yellow foci over the subpleural pulmonary parenchyma may be seen as a common incidental finding at post mortem in ferrets (see Plate 6). Histologically there are aggregates of lipid laden macrophages in the alveoli beneath the pleura. These lesions are superficial and cause no signs, but are often mistaken for metastasising neoplasms.

Respiratory syncytial virus

Ferrets can be infected with human respiratory syncytial virus. Minor histological changes may be seen, but it is not associated with any clinical signs.

Bovine rhinotracheitis virus

Ferrets can contract bovine rhinotracheitis virus, leading to an acute or chronic respiratory disease. There may be sneezing, coughing and anorexia. Natural outbreaks have not been reported, but this could occur in animals fed material from infected cattle.

Pneumocystis carinii

This organism, recently reclassified as a fungus, is found as a commensal in the lungs of many domestic and laboratory animals. Immunosuppression, for instance due to long-term corticosteroid administration, may lead to clinical disease. There is an interstitial pneumonia, with focal mononuclear cell infiltrates, parasitic cysts and trophozoites. Ferrets are fairly susceptible to corticosteroid induced pneumocystis pneumonia, so this should be considered as a differential in animals on long-term steroid therapy or those with hyperadrenocorticism which develop respiratory disease. Diagnosis may be made by examination of bronchial washings for trophozoites or by polymerase chain reaction. The condition can be treated with potentiated sulphonamides.

Intrathoracic masses

Primary or secondary neoplastic masses in the anterior thorax may lead to respiratory distress or dysphagia. The narrow thoracic inlet means that small masses will produce clinical signs at an early stage. In addition, these masses may result in a pleural effusion.

Mycoplasma mustelidae

This has been isolated from mink kits and ferrets but its importance is unknown.

Dirofilaria immitis (heartworms)

This may occur in imported animals (see Chapter 12).

Chlamydia

Ferrets are susceptible to intranasal infection with *Chlamydia*, and cases of pneumonitis and pneumonia have been reported. The lungs become firm, oedematous and plum coloured, with hyperplasia of the bronchiolar epithelium, oedema in the alveolar walls with a mononuclear infiltrate, and exudate containing mononuclear cells in the alveoli and bronchioles.

7 GASTROINTESTINAL DISEASES

Diseases of the mouth

Dental abnormalities are relatively common particularly in older ferrets, and are often an incidental finding on clinical examination. Occasionally, supernumerary teeth or dental malformations may be encountered: these usually require no treatment.

Fractures of the teeth are common, particularly in animals with a tendency to chew environmental objects, which often break the tips of the upper canines. Usually there are no clinical signs, but in cases where the pulp cavity is exposed, the condition may become painful and lead to anorexia. Such animals need root canal treatment or extraction of the affected tooth.

The presence of periodontal disease and dental calculus indicates that the diet is too soft, and is common in animals fed solely on moist food. It can also occur in animals which are immunosuppressed. If untreated, it can lead to gum disease and tooth decay, causing salivation and dysphagia. In severe cases, scale and polish the teeth under general anaesthesia. Recurrence can be reduced or prevented by the inclusion of small amounts of tough meat or biscuits in the diet.

Tooth root abscesses may be seen occasionally. Affected animals are often anorexic and may present with a swelling or draining tract over the zygomatic arch. Remove the affected tooth, giving appropriate antibiotics according to sensitivity, and leave the tract open to drain.

Neoplasms of the mouth are rare. Oral squamous cell carcinomas, fibrosarcomas, and salivary gland adenocarcinomas have been reported.

Salivary mucocoele

Ferrets have five pairs of salivary glands, the submandibular, sublingual, zygomatic, parotid and molar. Accumulation of saliva in the ducts of these glands produces a swelling in the corresponding area, commonly the commissures of the mouth or over the zygomatic arch (see Plate 7). Aspiration of the mass reveals clear viscous fluid, which may contain some blood. This condition may be treated successfully by marsupialisation: use a circular biopsy needle to create a stoma in the medial wall of the mass and remove the saliva. Alternatively, remove the gland completely taking care, particularly with the submandibular gland, not to damage the structures in the neck.

Diseases of the oesophagus

Oesophageal disease is uncommon in ferrets, although oesophageal foreign bodies occur rarely. Diagnose and treat foreign bodies as in the dog or cat.

Megaoesophagus occurs rarely in middle aged or older ferrets, although it has also been reported in young animals. It is usually acquired, but congenital megaoesophagus can occur and may remain subclinical or produce cyclical signs prior to becoming severe.

Aetiology and pathogenesis

The aetiology of megaoesophagus is unknown. Lead poisoning, myasthenia gravis, hypothyroidism, Addison's disease and nerve damage have all been suggested as possible causes, but often no cause is identified. There is dilatation of the intrathoracic oesophagus with an absence of motility, and there may be atrophy of the muscle layers or hyperkeratosis of the mucosal epithelium. The affected tissues can become colonised by yeasts, producing a lymphoid and neutrophil infiltration. Megaoesophagus leads to malnutrition, and can lead to secondary hepatic lipidosis or aspiration pneumonia.

Clinical signs

Affected animals are lethargic, with inappetence, anorexia, dysphagia, and weight loss. There may be regurgitation, with coughing or choking indicating aspiration of food material. Chronic cases may have aspiration pneumonia, with laboured breathing, dyspnoea and cyanosis.

Diagnosis

Diagnosis may be made on radiographic examination, which will reveal dilatation of the thoracic oesophagus. This can be confirmed using barium as a contrast medium: consider using an iodine based contrast medium in animals which have exhibited regurgitation to avoid the possibility of barium entering the lungs. Fluoroscopy or image intensification can be used to examine the motility of the oesophagus.

Once megaoesophagus has been confirmed, a broad based diagnostic approach is needed to investigate the underlying cause. Haematological, biochemical or serological tests may need to be performed to rule out the proposed causes of megaoesophagus outlined above.

Treatment and control

The prognosis for animals with megaoesophagus is poor, and treatment is usually unsuccessful. Supportive care, antibiotics, and gravity assisted feeding of small, semi-liquid meals several times daily may be beneficial. Gastrointestinal motility enhancers may also be of benefit but their effects have not been evaluated in ferrets. Try metoclopramide 0.2–1 mg/kg three to four times daily per os or by s.c. injection, or cisapride 0.5 mg/kg once to three times daily per os (recommended dose for dog). Euthanasia however is probably the best option for animals with this condition.

Gastritis, gastroduodenal ulceration and *Helicobacter mustelae*

Aetiology and pathogenesis

Inflammatory diseases of the stomach and proximal small intestine with or without ulceration may have several different causes, may be acute or chronic, and are often multifactorial. Foreign bodies, toxic ingestion, proliferative bowel disease (see below) or internal parasites are likely causes in younger animals, and in older animals neoplasia, uraemia, stress from chronic debilitating conditions, or prolonged treatment with ulcerogenic drugs, such as non-steroidal or steroidal anti-inflammatory drugs, must also be considered.

Gastroduodenal ulcers may be small pinpoint ulcers invisible to the naked eye, detected only by the presence of blood in the lumen of the organ, or large focal ulcers in the pyloric area which may erode into submucosal blood vessels. The precise mechanisms which allow ulcers to form are unknown, but stress may predispose to ulcer formation by reducing blood flow to the stomach, decreasing gastric cell turnover and gastric emptying, increasing gastric acid secretion, and reducing healing. Gastroduodenal ulcers cause anorexia and stress, leading to further development of the disease and a progressive deterioration in the animal's condition. Large ulcers which erode into blood vessels may result in a fatal gastric haemorrhage, which can cause death within minutes.

Helicobacter mustelae is a gram negative rod, similar to *H. pylori* in man, which is commonly found colonising the pyloric area of the stomach in up to 100% of animals from as young as five to six weeks. The organism causes a lymphoplasmacytic infiltration and loss of the glandular mucosa, leading to a mild gastritis, although clinical disease is rare. However, the disease can progress to produce ulceration and death, particularly at times of stress.

Clinical signs

Simple gastritis causes lethargy, anorexia and weight loss, vomiting, ptyalism, and tooth grinding (due to abdominal pain and nausea). Chronic cases are likely to be dehydrated. With gastroduodenal ulceration, there will also be melaena, peripheral lymphocytosis and regenerative anaemia. Tooth grinding and the presence of black tarry stools are highly suggestive of gastroduodenal ulceration.

Diagnosis

A detailed history and clinical examination will rule out many of the potential causes given above. Radiography is important to determine whether there is a foreign body, and a short period of fasting (two to four hours) will facilitate visualisation of gastric foreign bodies. Examination of vomitus or stools may be of use in diagnosing parasite infestations. *Helicobacter mustelae* can be diagnosed provisionally by exclusion, and confirmed by histopathology on biopsies of gastric mucosa, taken from the pyloric area. Examination of the stomach with a 3 mm fibre optic endoscope may be useful.

Treatment and control

Non-specific, supportive care may be all that is required in cases of simple gastritis. If the animal is not vomiting, provide frequent small meals of bland moist food high in carbohydrate and low in fibre. If the animal is vomiting, withhold food for 6–12 hours until vomiting ceases, then feed as above. Metoclopramide at 0.2–1 mg/kg may reduce vomiting, but its effects have not been fully evaluated in ferrets. Parenteral fluids and electrolytes may be needed if the animal has vomited copiously, and broad spectrum antibiotics can be given.

Specific therapy can be given if there is a definitive diagnosis. Foreign bodies should be removed under general anaesthesia.

Ulcers can be treated with bismuth subsalicylate, which is active against pepsin, at 0.25–1 ml/kg per os three to four times daily. Sucralfate is a cytoprotective agent and binds to the site of ulcers: give $\frac{1}{8}$ tablet four times daily. Cimetidine can be given to reduce gastric acid secretion, 10 mg/kg three times daily per os. All treatments need to be given for a minimum of seven to ten days, and it may take up to four weeks or more for ulcers to heal completely. In addition, the underlying cause should be investigated and treated.

Helicobacter mustelae infection can be treated using a combination of amoxycillin and metronidazole, both at 20 mg/kg twice daily per os, and bismuth subsalicylate 1 ml/kg twice daily. These need to be given for at least 14 days. *H. mustelae* may be sensitive to either antibiotic alone, but resistance develops rapidly unless they are given in combination. Other drugs which may be of use if the animal has bleeding ulcers are cimetidine (Tagamet, Pfizer) at 10 mg/kg three times daily, or famotidine (Pepcid, Morson) at 0.25 to 0.5 mg/kg once daily. Another regime which has been successful in eradicating *H. mustelae* is ranitidine bismuth citrate (Pylorid, Glaxo Wellcome) 24 mg/kg, and clarithromycin (Klaricid, Abbott) 12.5 mg/kg, both given per os three times daily. Recurrence is common, particularly at times of stress.

In all cases, stress is a major predisposing factor, so causes of stress should be removed from the environment. Gastritis and gastroduodenal ulceration both lead to anorexia and it is important to offer a bland, highly digestible diet to encourage the animal to eat and break the cycle which allows ulcers to form.

Foreign bodies

Intestinal foreign bodies are common in ferrets, because they are inquisitive and playful, though they are less common in the UK than the USA. In animals less than two years of age, the object is likely to be a plaything, such as a piece of rubber or cloth. In older animals, consider hairballs as well: these may be predisposed by chronic gastritis.

Clinical signs

Gastric foreign bodies may cause lethargy, intermittent inappetence, or diarrhoea with or without tarry stools. Vomiting is uncommon, although nausea can lead to ptyalism and face rubbing. These signs may progress to weakness and dehydration. Foreign bodies lodged at the pylorus can ulcerate through the stomach wall. Intestinal foreign bodies may cause sudden collapse and dehydration, with a painful abdomen.

Diagnosis

The diagnosis may be made on the history, clinical signs and a careful clinical examination. Palpate the abdomen carefully, although gastric foreign bodies can be hard to feel. Radiography is essential: fast the animal for a few hours beforehand to facilitate visualisation of gastric foreign bodies. The foreign body may or may not be visible, but there is likely to be gas in the stomach and segmental ileus, and contrast techniques are rarely needed. Perform full haematology on animals which have been ill for more than two to three days to check for anaemia and dehydration.

Treatment and control

Foreign bodies rarely pass unaided and removal under general anaesthesia is usually required (see Chapter 19). The animal should be stabilised first: parenteral fluids may be essential. Prevention of a recurrence may be achieved by 'ferret-proofing' the environment carefully, and by the regular use of a palatable cat laxative if necessary to reduce the formation of hairballs.

Vomiting

Vomiting is not as common in ferrets as it is in cats or dogs. Care must be taken to distinguish between regurgitation (oesophageal disorders) and vomiting (gastric disorders).

Aetiology

The most likely causes of vomiting are gastrointestinal foreign bodies, *Helicobacter mustelae*, and gastroenteritis. Mega-oesophagus causes regurgitation. It is important to be able to determine rapidly whether the treatment is likely to be medical or surgical.

Diagnosis and treatment

The diagnosis may be made on the history, and clinical examination: a foreign body may be palpable. Radiography, including the oeso-phagus, is a very important part of the diagnostic workup. If the radiograph is inconclusive, give the animal supportive care and repeat in 24 hours, by which time a foreign body may have become visible. An exploratory laparotomy may be indicated in any case, and a biopsy should be taken of the pyloric area to rule out *Heli-cobacter*. Following a diagnosis, treatment should be given as appropriate.

Eosinophilic gastroenteritis

Aetiology and pathogenesis

This is a rare condition which typically affects animals of six months to four years of age. The cause is unknown, but there may be an element of hypersensitivity to food or parasites, or an immunolo-gical component.

Clinical signs

There is weight loss and anorexia with chronic diarrhoea which may be bloody, and possibly vomiting. Clinical examination may reveal thickening of the intestines and enlargement of the mesenteric lymph nodes, and there may be swelling of the feet and ears. There is frequently a peripheral eosinophilia on haematology, and eosinophilic infiltration of the gastrointestinal tract and lymph nodes on histological examination.

Diagnosis

Other causes of diarrhoea should be ruled out before considering this disease. Diagnosis may be made on haematology or histopathology.

Treatment and control

Give supportive therapy, high calorie supplements and try hand feeding. Some success has been reported using ivermectin at 400 µg/kg, suggesting a parasitic component, although gastrointestinal parasites are rarely isolated in ferrets. Prednisone at 1.25–2.5 mg/kg orally once daily, reducing the dose weekly, may produce a resolution of clinical signs although treatment is often needed for the rest of the animal's life. Dietary manipulations may produce an improvement in clinical signs.

Proliferative bowel disease

Aetiology and pathogenesis

This disease affects ferrets mainly up to 14 months of age, usually males. It is associated with infection by an intracellular *Campylobacter* like organism (ICO), recently characterised as *Desulfovibrio* species. Infection is frequently complicated by other pathogens such as coccidia or *Campylobacter jejuni*, producing synergistic effects. Periods of disease may last up to six weeks, and recrudescence is common, particularly when the animal is stressed. In addition, the organism is often isolated from healthy animals. The organism(s) invades the mucosa of the colon, and occasionally also the small intestine, producing hyperplasia of the glandular epithelium, gross thickening of the intestinal wall and a 'cobblestone' appearance to the mucosa.

Clinical signs

The disease may begin as acute colitis, with tenesmus and pain on defaecation, profuse green diarrhoea, and flecks of blood. It can then progress to chronic diarrhoea, haematochezia, anorexia, weight loss, lethargy and rectal prolapse. Death may ensue if the animal becomes very dehydrated, or if the bowel perforates leading to peritonitis. Animals may also present with other signs, since they become susceptible to other diseases.

Diagnosis

The condition may be diagnosed on clinical signs, and confirmed by biopsy of the colon. Bacteria may be visible in the tissues with silver stains. The availability of primers for polymerase chain reaction (PCR) may aid in diagnosis.

Treatment and control

Treatment is often unrewarding, although supportive therapy may be helpful. Chloramphenicol at 50 mg/kg twice daily for two to three weeks may be effective: erythromycin and tetracyclines have both been tried to no effect.

Enteritis and diarrhoea

Enteritis in ferrets encompasses a spectrum of diseases from mild catarrhal enteritis to peracute infections causing toxaemia, hypovolaemic shock and sudden death. There can be disorders of motility leading to intussusception or rectal prolapse, which require surgical correction. Since the ferret's gut is short and the GI transit time is short, it is hard to distinguish between diarrhoeas of small and large intestinal origin.

Aetiology

Non-infectious causes include dietary indiscretion, foreign bodies, eosinophilic gastroenteritis and hairballs.

Many infectious agents can produce diarrhoea, including proliferative bowel disease and canine distemper virus. *Salmonella* infection may occur in animals fed uncooked meat or poultry products. Animals may be symptomless carriers, or it may cause bloody diarrhoea and endotoxic shock. It can also cause conjunctivitis and undulating fever, with dehydration, anorexia, and malaise. The disease is very contagious and has implications for human health, so strict attention must be paid to hygiene and disinfection. Aggressive supportive care and antibiotic therapy should be given according to sensitivity, and the source identified and excluded from the diet.

Rotavirus infection is associated with diarrhoea in kits four to six weeks old. There is high morbidity, and mortality. In adults, the disease is mild, producing green mucoid diarrhoea. Treat with supportive therapy.

Mycobacterium bovis and *M. avium* have both been isolated from ferrets where the animals have been given raw meat or poultry or unpasteurised dairy products. There may be chronic weight loss with vomiting and diarrhoea. If the history is suggestive, exploratory laparotomy can be performed to take biopsies to look for acid fast organisms. Treatment is not recommended: affected animals should be culled.

Campylobacter jejuni may be isolated from normal ferrets and in those with diarrhoea and enterocolitis, and may be isolated from cases of proliferative bowel disease although its clinical significance is unsure. There may also be zoonotic implications.

Epizootic catarrhal enteritis has been identified recently in the USA, and is a disease with high morbidity and low mortality, possibly caused by a coronavirus. The animal has profuse green slimy diarrhoea, which may progress to ulceration and bloody faeces. Give aggressive supportive therapy, and try bismuth (0.25–1 ml/kg per os three to four times daily) and loperamide (Imodium syrup, Janssen) at 100–200 µg/kg.

Diagnosis

The diagnosis of enteritis depends on the severity and duration of clinical signs. Take a detailed history, and determine the vaccination history. Fresh faecal samples can be taken for culture and parasite analysis.

Treatment and control

In mild cases, supportive care and dietary management will be sufficient. Overtly ill animals need to be hospitalised and given aggressive supportive therapy. Following a detailed diagnostic workup, specific therapy can be given. Motility modifiers should not be given unless the diagnosis has been confirmed.

Other gastrointestinal diseases

Neoplasia

Gastrointestinal neoplasia is not common in ferrets, and tumours are most often found in the parenchymal organs (liver, pancreas) and intestine. The most common tumours are primary tumours or metastases in the liver, such as lymphosarcomas or insulinomas, or lymphomas of the mesenteric lymph nodes. Hepatic neoplasms frequently present with ascites. Fibrosarcomas of the oral mucosa present as firm smooth masses which grow rapidly to cover the teeth. Aggressive resection may give temporary alleviation of signs but the prognosis is poor. Pyloric adenocarcinomas may present with signs similar to those of a gastric foreign body, and removal of the affected area may produce an improvement for a prolonged period. In man, infection with *Helicobacter pylori* has been implicated in the aetiology of gastric adenocarcinoma, and this may also be the case in ferrets with *H. mustelae*. Other neoplasms which have been reported include hepatic haemangiosarcomas, bile duct cystadenomas, and cholangiomas arising from the bile duct epithelium, which are sometimes encountered as incidental findings in older animals. Clinical signs depend on the location of the tumour, and suggested treatments include debulking surgery and chemo-therapy. The prognosis is poor however, unless the entire tumour can be resected.

Rectal prolapse

This is usually secondary to other diseases such as proliferative bowel disease, *Campylobacter*, parasite infestations and non-specific diarrhoea. Most cases resolve spontaneously once the underlying problem has gone. If necessary, a temporary purse string suture can be used for two to three days, or in chronic cases the anus can be tightened by removing a wedge of skin.

Anal gland disease

Infection, impaction, abscessation and neoplasia of the anal glands may all occur, producing pain on defaecation, with ribbon like stools. Palpate the area carefully, for uni- or bilateral swellings (see Plate 8). In cases of infection, flush under general anaesthesia and treat with antibiotics. In chronic cases the anal sacs may be removed surgically, but this often results in incontinence. Surgical debulking of neoplasms may be attempted, but the prognosis is poor and again faecal incontinence may result.

Parasites

Unusually for a carnivore, the ferret does not appear to be a natural or intermediate host for any nematode or cestode. If an infestation is found, it is usually described as 'accidental'. They can become infected by the same ascarids and tapeworms as cats and dogs, and may be treated as cats. Occasionally, coccidia or *Giardia* spp. may be seen. Coccidia appear to be asymptomatic and self-limiting, although they could act synergistically with other organisms, producing pathology. Coccidia have been found coinfecting with *Desulfovibrio* in cases of proliferative bowel disease.

8 MUSCULOSKELETAL AND NEUROLOGIC DISEASES

Posterior paresis, ataxia and seizures

Aetiology and pathogenesis

Posterior paresis and ataxia are relatively common presenting features in ferrets, and may have many causes. Any disease causing generalised weakness may appear to present as posterior paresis, since the hindlimb muscles are often more affected than the others. Diseases which produce abdominal pain such as cystic calculi or splenomegaly may cause alterations in gait which mimic hindlimb weakness. Metabolic diseases causing posterior paresis or ataxia include hypocalcaemia in nursing jills, thiamine deficiency, and hypoglycaemia secondary to insulinoma or anorexia. Cardiac disease, bone marrow depression, anaemia or toxins may cause CNS depression, ataxia and weakness. Other aetiologies which have been associated with similar signs include systemic mycoses, toxoplasmosis, eosinophilic granulomas, distemper virus infection and copper toxicosis.

Primary neurological disorders resulting in hindlimb paresis include spinal trauma, intervertebral disc disease, hemivertebrae, myeloma, chordomas, and Aleutian disease virus infection (see below).

Seizures are uncommon, but may occur if there is hypocalcaemia, hypoglycaemia, toxaemia or central nervous system infection, trauma or neoplasia. Idiopathic epilepsy has not been reported in the ferret.

Clinical signs

The animal may present with abducted hindlimbs, or a frog-legged appearance (see Plate 9). The hindlegs are incoordinated, and the body may lose its curved appearance as the animal is unable to flex the spine as much as usual. The withdrawal and placing reflexes may be absent, and the animal may be incontinent. Often, the animal remains bright and alert and otherwise normal.

Diagnosis

The many different possible causes can be distinguished by a thorough clinical examination and diagnostic workup. Take a detailed history to determine the animal's reproductive status and disease status of the colony, and to exclude the possibility of toxic ingestion. During the clinical examination, check for cardiac dysrhythmias and palpate the abdomen carefully. Perform a neurological and orthopaedic examination, looking for normal or abnormal reflexes, spinal pain or hyperaesthesia. Take blood to check for the glucose level, and perform complete haematology, biochemistry, and serology for Aleutian disease or distemper. Take x-rays of the spinal column, chest and abdomen: myelography can be useful for determining if there is intervertebral disc disease. This can be performed in the anaesthetised animal in sternal recumbency through the lumbar approach. Place a 20 or 22G spinal needle through the space between L5 and L6 under aseptic conditions with the animal's hindlegs extended forwards to open up the intervertebral space. Alternatively, the needle can be placed in the atlanto-occipital joint. This can also be useful for obtaining a sample of cerebrospinal fluid.

Treatment and control

Specific treatment depends on the diagnosis. Non-specific supportive therapy, cage rest and prednisolone may be effective in cases of disc disease, or viral myelitis. However, recurrence is common and the prognosis is then guarded.

Aleutian disease

Aetiology and pathogenesis

Aleutian disease is caused by a parvovirus, and is so named because Aleutian mink are particularly susceptible to it. Mink develop an immune complex glomerulonephritis, which is often fatal. Ferrets have an antigenically distinct strain of virus, which may have originated from the mink strain. Some surveys in the USA have suggested that up to 40% of ferrets may be infected. Welchman, Oxenham and Done (1993) found 8.5% of ferrets to have antibody in a survey of pet and working ferrets in southern England, and in another institution, 25 of 40 ferrets tested positive in one colony whereas no infected animals were found in another colony of 40 animals housed in a different building and using a different supplier (author). Following infection, the virus replicates in liver and spleen, there is persistent viraemia and a massive ineffectual immune response. By day 63 post infection there may be hypergammaglobulinaemia and immune complex formation, leading to lymphocytic, plasmacytic infiltration of multiple organ systems. Clinical signs depend on the organs most affected: there may be glomerulonephritis, vasculitis, thyroiditis, perivascular lymphocyte cuffing, lymphadenopathy and hepatosplenomegaly. Frequently there is central nervous involvement, with a non-suppurative encephalomyelitis.

The virus can be spread both vertically and horizontally, via contact with infected secretions and excretions, although the transmission rate appears to be low.

Clinical signs

Often, there are no clinical signs at all. In other cases there may be posterior paralysis and ataxia which may progress to quadriplegia, chronic progressive wasting, cachexia, melaena, ill thrift, poor reproductive performance, collapse and sudden death. Other animals may have repeated episodes of posterior paresis but remain bright and alert and otherwise unaffected. Clinical disease in subclinical cases can be precipitated by stress factors. Infection may also increase the animal's susceptibility to other diseases, such as proliferative bowel disease or lymphoid neoplasia, and secondary bacterial infections. Animals between eight months and seven years have been affected, and the signs may develop over 24 hours or progress over several months.

Diagnosis

If Aleutian disease is suspected, a diagnosis can be made by counter-immunoelectrophoresis (CIEP) on a sample of plasma, which can be done by Harlan Seralab, Dodgeford Lane, Belton, Loughborough, Leics. This can be taken simply by clipping a toenail in the conscious animal and collecting the blood into a heparinised capillary tube. It may be necessary to test two samples taken 21 days apart, since seroconversion may take this long. Another useful diagnostic indicator is a raised gamma globulin level in plasma. Histopathology from clinically affected animals may reveal lymphocyte and plasma cell infiltration of the meninges, and inflammatory and degenerative changes in the spinal cord, including perivascular cuffing, mononuclear infiltrates and focal malacia. However, there may be no histopathological changes, and there are no consistent haematological changes.

Treatment and control

No specific treatment is available. Animals may respond to supportive therapy, corticosteroids and antibiotics although they will remain infected and present a risk to other animals. Culling of infected animals is recommended. Since the transmission rate is low, it is possible to test individual animals, and cull those testing positive. Two tests at least three weeks apart should allow the virus to be eradicated from a colony.

Botulism

Aetiology and pathogenesis

Ferrets are very susceptible to the toxin produced by *Clostridium botulinum*, particularly type C but also types A and B. The organisms are strict anaerobes, and will only multiply and produce toxin under the correct conditions, typically in decaying meat and animal carcases. Ingestion of pre-formed botulinum toxin in spoiled food results in blockage of the release of acetylcholine at the neuromuscular junction, leading to flaccid paralysis.

Clinical signs

Signs appear approximately 96 hours after the ingestion of toxin, although animals may be found dead as soon as 48 hours after exposure to the toxin. The animal becomes incoordinated, with paresis or generalised flaccid paralysis, and there may be dysphagia and ptyalism. Death occurs due to paralysis of the respiratory muscles.

Diagnosis

Signs of flaccid paralysis in several animals at once with a history of ingestion of spoiled food is indicative of botulism. The diagnosis can be confirmed by demonstration of toxin in food or ingesta.

Treatment and control

Reduce further absorption of toxin by gavaging with adsorbants such as activated charcoal. The prognosis in affected animals is poor, although occasionally animals recover without treatment.

The condition may be prevented by feeding a commercially prepared diet, which does not contain 'fresh' meat likely to become spoiled. If raw mince is to be fed, use it as soon as possible after purchase, and remove any which is not eaten. The causative organism is a natural contaminant of wild bird carcases, so avoid giving these to ferrets. Annual vaccination with type C toxoid may protect against the disease.

Other diseases with neurological or musculoskeletal signs

Canine distemper virus

This may cause neurological signs in the late stages of the disease, and central nervous system involvement has been noted from 12 days post infection. There may be hyperexcitability, salivation, muscle tremors, seizures, coma and death. This disease is discussed in Chapter 6.

Hypoglycaemia

This occurs secondary to pancreatic insulinomas, and may result in intermittent episodes of abnormal behaviour, weakness, ataxia and tremors, paraplegia, and collapse. Blood glucose levels will be low, and insulin may be high, up to $40\,\mu U/ml$. If the blood glucose is below $60\,mg/dl$, intravenous dextrose should be given to effect and exploratory surgery planned to look for insulinomas. This is covered in Chapter 9, Endocrine Diseases.

Rabies

Ferrets do not appear to be very active vectors of rabies, but it may occur in animals imported from rabies endemic areas. At present, ferrets are required to enter six months of rabies quarantine on arrival in the UK. Both furious and dumb forms of rabies are recognised in ferrets. The initial signs are anxiety and lethargy, but it may present as a progressive posterior paralysis.

Nutritional problems
(see also Chapter 14)

Thiamine deficiency

This may occur in animals fed diets high in eggs or raw fish, which have high thiaminase activity. Signs are most often seen in the 8–12 week age group, and include anorexia, hind limb weakness and convulsions. Death may follow within two to three days. Outbreaks have been seen in kits aged two to three weeks on a farm, who were fed a diet high in uncooked fish. The animals developed anorexia, depression, malaise, weight loss and greasy coats, and died within 24 hours. Injections of vitamin B-complex, 5 mg daily for three days, may produce a resolution.

Zinc toxicity

Ferrets are very susceptible to zinc toxicity. There may be lethargy, anaemia and hind limb weakness, leading to renal and hepatic failure. There is no treatment and the prognosis is poor. Care should be taken not to use galvanised water and food bowls for ferrets.

Osteodystrophy

Feeding an all meat diet leads to calcium deficiency and osteody-strophy. Animals between 6 and 12 weeks are most affected. They may present with a seal-like gait, with abducted front legs, and the bones are soft and deformed. Often, there is sudden death of several kits in a litter which otherwise look well nourished. Diagnosis can be made on clinical signs and radiography. Correct the diet of affected animals, or use balanced mineral and vitamin supplements such as Pet-Cal (Pfizer) or SA-37 (Intervet). Recovered animals may be permanently deformed (see Plate 10).

Fractures

Ferrets involved in road accidents or other trauma may present with fractures. Treat these as for cats: conservative management may be sufficient, or surgical treatment may be necessary. Ferrets will tolerate amputation of a limb reasonably well.

Neoplasia

Neoplasms of the central nervous system in ferrets have been reported very rarely, and reports of skeletal neoplasms are also rare. Osteomas of the skull and chordomas (neoplasms arising from the remnant of the notochord, often at the tip of the tail) have been noted most commonly. A synovial sarcoma affecting the stifle joint, a fibrosarcoma of the femur, and a chondroma of the tail have also been reported. Other tumours which may be encountered uncommonly are leiomyomas arising from the smooth muscle of blood vessel walls. Removal of these lesions can be curative.

Osteomas usually present as firm, dense bony masses arising from the zygomatic arch or parietal bone. These are benign, but may cause clinical signs due to pressure on surrounding tissues. Diagnosis is made by radiography. Surgical removal can be curative if the tumour is in a site amenable to resection.

Chordomas usually present as lobulated, firm ulcerated masses at the tip of the tail, although they have been described in the cervical region. They are locally invasive and destroy the vertebral body and adjacent tissues. Those located at the tail tip may be removed; several vertebrae proximal to the lesion should also be resected. Although potentially malignant, chordomas rarely metastasise and resection will be curative.

Cataracts

This condition (see Plate 11) is thought to be common although there are few reports in the literature. One report showed that in a population of ferrets, more than 46% had lens opacities at 11–12 months (Miller *et al.*, 1993). These were of several types, and many were progressive, leading eventually to blindness. The development of cataracts may be influenced by congenital and genetic factors, and there may be dietary components. A high level of rancid fat in the diet could lead to the formation of oxyradicals which aggregate lens crystalline proteins. Deficiencies in vitamin E or protein can lead to the formation of cataracts in other species, and may be a factor in ferrets.

Congenital neural tube defects

These are among the most common congenital defects. Abnormalities range from anencephaly, cranioschisis (external opening of the skull), craniorachischisis (opening of skull and spinal cord with loss of cerebral tissue), and spina bifida, to fusion or deformation of vertebrae.

Creutzfeld Jakob Disease

A transmissible spongiform encephalopathy has been passed to ferrets experimentally. There are no reports of naturally occurring prion disease in ferrets.

Larva Migrans

Two young ferrets which presented with weakness and circling prior to death were found to have suppurative encephalitis associated with aberrant parasite migration.

References

Miller, P.E., Marlar, A.B. and Dubielzig, R.R. (1993) Cataracts in a laboratory colony of ferrets. *Laboratory Animal Science*, **43**(6), pp. 562–8.

Welchman, D. de B., Oxenham, M. and Done, S.H. (1993) Aleutian disease in domestic ferrets: diagnostic findings and survey results. *Veterinary Record*, **132**, pp. 479–84.

9 ENDOCRINE DISEASES

Hyperoestrogenism

Aetiology and pathogenesis

Jills are induced ovulators, and require vigorous, prolonged copulation to stimulate ovulation. Jills which are not bred may remain in oestrus for the duration of the natural breeding season, normally March to September in the UK. The high levels of endogenous oestrogens produced may lead to progressive suppression of the bone marrow. If this occurs, the production of all blood cells is affected, leading to leucopenia, thrombocytopenia and aplastic anaemia. All jills will develop at least a mild anaemia during oestrus at some point, and up to 50% of jills with prolonged oestrus will develop aplastic anaemia. In addition, there may be liver dysfunction leading to a coagulopathy of dual origin, and increased susceptibility to secondary bacterial diseases due to the leucopenia.

Clinical signs

The signs are combined with those of oestrus. There may be a bilaterally symmetrical alopecia on the ventral abdomen and tail, weight loss, enlarged vulva (see Figure 1.2), and a serous or mucopurulent vaginal discharge. This may progress to anorexia, depression and lethargy, and generalised weakness. Other signs associated with depression of the bone marrow will be present, such as pale mucous membranes and a systolic murmur associated with anaemia, and secondary bacterial infections due to leucopenia. A coagulopathy associated with the thrombocytopenia and liver dysfunction will lead to petechiae, ecchymoses, melaena, and haemorrhages. Subdural haematomas may lead to posterior paralysis, and death is often due to haemorrhage, particularly if the platelet count falls below 20 000 per mm^3. This is seen most often in animals which have been in oestrus for more than two months.

Diagnosis

The diagnosis can be made on history and clinical signs, and confirmed by haematology. A PCV of less than 20% and concurrent depression of all blood cell series in an oestrous female are highly indicative of hyperoestrogenism. There may be some nucleated red blood cells, but the marrow response is insufficient to maintain adequate levels of red cells. Post mortem examination of animals which die reveals pale tissues with haemorrhages. There may be frank blood in the intestines, and suppurative infections such as pyometra are common. Histopathology reveals hypocellularity of the bone marrow.

Treatment and control

Treatment is aimed at removing the source of oestrogens, and ovariohysterectomy is the fastest way to achieve this, although initial treatment must be dictated by the PCV. If the animal has a low platelet count and PCV of 15–25%, give a blood transfusion prior to the procedure (see page 163, Chapter 18, Sedation, Anaesthesia and Analgesia). In less severe cases where the PCV is 25% or above, hormone treatments can be used to induce ovulation. Give either human chorionic gonadotrophin (HCG) (Chorulon, Intervet, 20–100 units i.m.) or proligestone (Delvosteron, Intervet, 0.5 ml s.c.) ten days after the onset of oestrus, and ovulation will occur within two days. The vulva will soften within three to four days and all signs of oestrus will then abate within three to four weeks. Supportive treatments such as anabolic steroids, B vitamins, a high calorie diet, fluids and antibiotics may be given as necessary, and it may take up to four months for the anaemia to resolve. Once the jill is no longer in heat, perform an ovariohysterectomy.

The prognosis for ferrets with hyperoestrogenism depends on the length of time the animal has been in oestrus and exposed to high oestrogen levels beforehand, so prompt treatment is essential. The prognosis can also be determined by the packed cell volume (PCV) on presentation. If the PCV is 25% or above, the prognosis is good. If it is 15–25%, the prognosis is guarded, and if it is below 15%, the outlook is poor and very intensive therapy will be required if the animal is to have a chance of survival. This may include multiple blood transfusions over a period of months, force feeding, anabolic steroid injections and vitamin supplementation.

To prevent a recurrence, do not permit oestrous females to remain in heat for longer than one month. There are several options for jills which are not to be bred. Ovariohysterectomy in females at six to eight months of age is the recommended method (see Chapter 19). Alternatively, running a group of intact females with a vasectomised male (or hobble) will result in induction of ovulation and a pseudopregnancy lasting about 42 days before the jill returns to oestrus. This has the advantage that the jills can still be bred in the future. Ovulation can be induced by stimulation of the vagina using a sterilised thermometer or similar instrument, although this may need to be performed for a prolonged period and combined with grasping the scruff of the neck to simulate natural mating, and is often ineffective. Hormone treatments can also be used as above, although these need repeating each season. As a preventive measure, dose jills exposed to natural daylight with proligestone in the last week in March. This will usually postpone oestrus until the following breeding season, although in about 10% of jills a repeat injection will be needed later in the same season. Proligestone can also be given to jills which are already in oestrus, and signs will abate within 10–11 days. However, if it is given to pregnant jills, it may result in delayed parturition and mummification of the fetuses, since it persists for longer than the normal gestation period (see Kluth, 1993). Proligestone may cause pain on injection. HCG leads to a pseudopregnancy lasting 40–50 days, then the jill will return to oestrus. Occasionally, two injections ten days apart will be required to produce a resolution of signs.

Ovarian remnants

Spayed females which show signs of oestrus are likely to have either an ovarian remnant or an adrenal tumour. These can be differentiated by response to treatment with proligestone or HCG: ovarian remnants respond and the signs of oestrus will abate, whereas adrenal tumours do not. Perform an exploratory laparotomy to remove the ovarian remnant and prevent hyperoestrogenism.

Insulinoma

Aetiology and pathogenesis

Functional tumours of the β-cells of the islets of Langerhans are reportedly common in ferrets in the USA. These may be adenomas, but are often adenocarcinomas. They produce excess levels of insulin, increasing glucose uptake by the cells, and inhibiting gluconeogenesis and glycogenolysis, causing hypoglycaemia. The disease may have an acute or chronic course. Animals between three and eight years old may be affected, but it is particularly seen in animals of four to five years of age. There have been no reported cases in the UK. The reason for this is unknown, but the high incidence seen in the USA may be related to the intensive breeding and genetic selection which occur there.

Clinical signs

The clinical signs depend on the rate of decline of the blood sugar level, and the level and duration of hypoglycaemia. Neurological signs occur due to the effects of low blood sugar on the CNS. Animals may present with disorientation, apparent blindness, ptyalism, generalised or hind leg weakness, or muscle twitches. There may be seizures in response to stimuli or excitement. Initially, neurological signs are intermittent, episodes lasting from minutes to hours. Prolonged or severe hypoglycaemia can lead to hypoxia causing brain damage. If the blood glucose level falls very rapidly, the release of catecholamines may lead to tachycardia, hypothermia, tremor, nervousness or irritability as presenting signs. Alternatively, there may be a gradual onset of weakness, hind leg ataxia and lethargy over several weeks.

Occasionally, there are no clinical signs, and pancreatic nodules are discovered during abdominal surgery performed for other reasons. It is not uncommon to find insulinomas in animals with concurrent adrenal or lymphoid neoplasms, or cardiomyopathy, so a thorough clinical examination is needed to rule these out.

Diagnosis

The clinical signs are suggestive, and the diagnosis can be confirmed by lowered blood glucose levels. It may be necessary to take more than one sample, or fast the animal for a short period (between four and six hours) to be certain. Use a test strip to measure blood glucose level, since the volume of any blood sample is likely to be small, and dividing samples between EDTA, heparin and oxalate/fluoride tubes will not always be feasible. Measurement of the insulin level is also useful. A raised insulin level (from normal up to 2000 pmol/l) in conjunction with a low blood glucose level (less than 70 mg/dl) is highly suggestive of insulinoma. Exploratory laparotomy will confirm the presence of nodules in the pancreas.

Treatment and control

Treatment may be medical or surgical. Medical treatment is recommended for ferrets with intercurrent diseases or those over six years of age. Treatment with prednisone (0.5–2 mg/kg twice daily per os) and/or diazoxide (5–10 mg/kg twice daily per os) may control the hypoglycaemia by increasing gluconeogenesis and inhibiting insulin release respectively, although there is no effect on the progression of the disease. Give frequent small high protein meals avoiding sugary foods (which stimulate insulin release), with no periods of fasting. Medical treatment can control the signs of the disease for as long as 18 months.

Surgical removal of the tumour tissue is recommended for younger animals, and if concurrent adrenal disease is suspected. This is usually a palliative measure, slowing but not arresting the progression of the disease. Details of the procedure can be found in Chapter 19, Common Surgical Procedures. Following removal of the tumours the animal will require fluids, antibiotics and frequent meals. Treatment with prednisolone (0.2 mg twice daily) and diazoxide (5 mg twice daily) may still be needed to control clinical signs.

If an animal presents during a hypoglycaemic crisis, give liquid glucose or honey per os using a syringe. If the animal has collapsed, rub glucose on the gingiva, taking care not to put fingers into the animal's mouth if it is likely to have a seizure. If there is no response, a bolus of 50% dextrose may be given *slowly* i.v. until the animal responds; typically 0.5–2 ml is needed. Care must be taken not to give this too fast, or the insulinoma will be stimulated to produce more insulin, producing a worsening of the clinical signs. It may be necessary to give an infusion of 5% dextrose over a prolonged period in severe cases, and diazepam (1–2 mg i.v. to effect) may be needed to control seizures. Once the animal is conscious, return to management as above.

Metastasis of insulinomas to other organs is rare, but local recurrence is likely and the overall prognosis is guarded.

Adrenal-related endocrinopathy

Aetiology and pathogenesis

This occurs if there is a functional adrenal adenoma or adeno-carcinoma, and could occur due to adrenal hyperplasia secondary to pituitary neoplasia, although this has not been reported. One or both adrenals may be affected: in unilateral cases it is often the left adrenal which is involved, both glands are affected in approximately 15% of cases. Adrenal tumours rarely metastasise, but may be locally invasive, eroding into the vena cava. The disease is most often seen in animals of two years of age or older, and is apparently more common in females. It is particularly common in the USA, but rare in the UK. Possible reasons for this include early neutering (at five to six weeks of age) and the tendency to keep animals indoors under unnatural lighting – conditions which occur in the USA, whereas in the UK animals are usually kept outdoors in natural lighting conditions and often remain entire.

The diseased adrenals produce increased levels of steroid hormones, which may be glucocorticoids, but are more commonly androgens, oestradiol or 17-hydroxyprogesterone, hence the term adrenal-related endocrinopathy, to distinguish this condition from hyperadrenocorticism (Cushing's syndrome).

Clinical signs

The overproduction of glucocorticoids is rare, so signs of Cushing's syndrome are uncommon (polydipsia and polyuria, muscle weakness, thinning of the skin and susceptibility to other diseases). The secretion of high levels of androgens and oestrogens leads to cutaneous, reproductive and behavioural changes in affected animals. Approximately 90% of cases develop a bilaterally symmetrical alopecia which begins at the tailhead and progresses forwards. This begins in the winter or spring, and may leave the animal completely bald. It is common for the fur to regrow in the autumn. The condition is often pruritic, with or without alopecia.

Females develop vulval swelling in 70% of cases, and may develop a vaginal discharge or pyometra. Males may develop dysuria or stranguria, due to hyperplasia in the region of the prostate or paraurethral cysts which fill with secretory material and keratin. These may be palpated as variably sized fluctuant cysts in the area of the bladder neck. They may also develop swelling in the mammary tissue.

In both sexes, there may be increased mounting behaviour and aggression, and males may show increased marking behaviour or feminisation.

Bone marrow suppression is rarely seen in cases of adrenal-related endocrinopathy, but may occur in long standing cases leading to anaemia, petechiation and other signs associated with hyperoestrogenism.

It may be possible to palpate the enlarged adrenals, particularly the left gland which lies cranial to the kidney in a fat pad.

Diagnosis

Diagnosis can usually be made on history and clinical signs, which are highly suggestive, particularly if there is an enlarged vulva in an ovariohysterectomised female. Haematology, biochemistry and radiography are usually inconclusive. Increased levels of androgens and oestrogens (see Table 9.1) are indicative of adrenal neoplasia or hyperplasia. These hormones are present at almost negligible levels in neutered animals. If oestradiol alone is elevated, the cause may be ovarian.

Table 9.1 Steroid hormone levels in cases of adrenal neoplasia (after Rosenthal, 1997).

Hormone	Normal	Diseased
Androstenedione (nmol/l)	6.6	67
Dehydroepiandrosterone sulphate (μmol/l)	0.01	0.03
Oestradiol (pmol/l)	106	167
17-hydroxyprogesterone (nmol/l)	0.4	3.2

To differentiate adrenal neoplasia from hyperoestrogenism, give the animal 100 i.u. human chorionic gonadotrophin in two doses seven to ten days apart, or proligestone 0.5 ml s.c. once. If the aetiology is ovarian, the vulval swelling will regress.

Rarely, animals may present with signs consistent with Cushing's syndrome, in which case there will be a stress leucogram and elevated cortisol levels. In these animals, an ACTH stimulation test and low dose dexamethasone suppression test can be used to confirm the diagnosis. For an ACTH stimulation test, take a baseline blood sample, then administer 1 unit/kg synthetic ACTH i.m. Take a second blood sample 30–60 minutes later. If the cortisol level rises by more than 40% of baseline level, this is indicative of Cushing's syndrome.

For the low dose dexamethasone suppression test, give 0.1 mg/kg dexamethasone i.v. after taking a baseline blood sample. Further samples are taken after four, six and eight hours. In the normal animal, the cortisol level will fall by approximately 27% of the baseline value at six to eight hours post dexamethasone. In cases of hyperadrenocorticism, the fall is much less. In pituitary dependent hyperadrenocorticism, there may be some suppression at four hours with a return to normal at eight hours. However, this is very rare in ferrets.

A definitive diagnosis may be made by biopsy of the adrenal tissue.

Treatment and control

Before beginning treatment, it is important to confirm the diagnosis and rule out other intercurrent diseases. Treatment for adrenal-related endocrinopathy may be medical or surgical. Surgical treatment is most effective, and is preferred for animals less than five years of age and for those which present with stranguria. Perform an exploratory laparotomy, making a thorough check of all abdominal organs and both adrenal glands. The adrenals may be found in the fat pads cranial to the kidneys. Normally, they measure three to five mm in length: if they are larger than this they are likely to be diseased. If only one adrenal is involved, remove it. If both are diseased, it is best to remove the left gland and 'shell out' the right, since the anatomy makes total removal of the right adrenal difficult. See Chapter 19 for further details. Post operatively, the animal may require supplementary corticosteroids if there has been total removal of both glands. Hair regrowth usually begins within two to six weeks, although it may be delayed until the next seasonal moult.

Medical treatment may be given in older animals which are poor candidates for surgery. Mitotane can be given at 50 mg per os once daily for seven days, then every three days for maintenance. The success of treatment can be monitored by clinical signs, but it tends to be rather unpredictable.

Paraurethral cysts can be removed or drained, although they usually regress spontaneously after adrenalectomy (see Chapters 13 and 19).

Diabetes mellitus

This is very rare but has been reported in ferrets. It may also occur secondarily to surgery for insulinoma. Common clinical signs include polydipsia, polyuria, and weight loss with increased appetite. The animal may be lethargic, particularly if there is concurrent ketoacidosis. Diagnosis may be confirmed by demonstration of a fasting hyperglycaemia (above 400 mg/dl), with glycosuria, reduced plasma insulin levels and possibly ketones in the urine.

Treatment may be unrewarding. It is important to establish a routine with set amounts of food given at regular times. Monitor the animal's food and water intake and activity. If the blood glucose level at presentation is above 300 mg/dl, try giving an intermediate acting insulin preparation (such as isophane or NPH) at 0.1 unit twice daily: this may need to be adjusted until the animal responds appropriately. Up to 5 units insulin may be needed daily. Check the blood and urine glucose levels, and discharge the animal when the blood glucose level has fallen below 200 mg/dl. The owner can be shown how to give subcutaneous insulin injections, and supplied with urine test sticks. It may be worth trying Ultralente insulin, which gives the option for once daily dosing.

Diabetes which is secondary to insulinoma surgery usually resolves spontaneously within a few weeks without the need for insulin treatment. Spontaneous cases however have proved difficult to manage, and the prognosis is guarded.

Thyroid disease

Thyroid disease is reported vary rarely in ferrets. Thyroiditis associated with Aleutian disease has been reported but causes no clinical signs. Thyroid adenocarcinoma has been reported rarely, and causes weight loss and alopecia, with a swelling in the ventral neck.

REFERENCES

Kluth, G.A. (1993) Oestrus control in ferrets. *Veterinary Record*, **133**:10, p. 252.

Rosenthal, K. (1997) Endocrine diseases: Part II. In: E.V. Hillyer and K.E. Quesenberry (eds), *Ferrets, Rabbits, and Rodents: Clinical Medicine and Surgery*. W.B. Saunders, Philadelphia, pp. 91–98.

10 DERMATOLOGIC DISEASES

As in other species, many systemic diseases in the ferret manifest with skin changes, and failure to groom is often an early sign of ill health. Skin conditions alert ferret owners to problems, causing them to seek veterinary advice early in the course of a disease, and so they can be common presenting signs.

A thorough and systematic approach is needed to investigate and diagnose skin conditions. It is important to take a full history, including details of diet and food intake, breeding activity and behaviour. Take time to assess the animal's behaviour when it is undisturbed, looking for evidence of scratching, abnormal grooming or rubbing of body parts. Check the environment the animal is kept in, paying particular attention to the bedding material, diet and hygiene, and enquire as to the health of in-contact animals. This information will assist in drawing up a list of differential diagnoses.

Since skin diseases are often secondary to systemic diseases, it is important to perform a thorough clinical examination, following this up with appropriate diagnostic tests. These may include general tests such as radiography, ultrasonography, blood or urine samples, as well as microscopy, bacterial or fungal culture on skin and hair samples. It may be necessary to sedate the animal to perform some of these tests.

A guide to diagnosis of conditions affecting the skin can be found in Figure 10.1.

Infectious diseases

Bacterial skin diseases

Fighting and biting injuries, which occur particularly in the breeding season and during mating, can result in superficial or deep skin infections, abscesses, or cellulitis. These are commonly caused by *Staphylococcus spp*, *Streptococcus spp*, *Pasteurella spp* or *Corynebacterium spp*. For superficial infections and abrasions, clipping and cleaning the area with topical antiseptic are usually all that is required. Occasionally, systemic antibiotics will be needed.

Deeper infections in the form of abscesses may develop following fighting injuries or penetration of the oral or oesophageal mucosa by sharp objects such as hay or bones. Occasionally, fragments of hay may be found within these abscesses, which are often located under the chin or in the mammary area (see Plate 12). Drain and flush abscesses under general anaesthesia, and give systemic antibiotics as appropriate following bacterial culture and sensitivity. Swabs for bacteriology should be taken from the wall of the abscess, not from the pus in the centre since this is likely to be sterile. Abscesses are sometimes very thick walled and may consist of several interconnecting pockets of purulent material within a fibrous capsule. These are best removed under general anaesthesia within their capsule, since otherwise it is difficult to establish drainage and recurrence is common. Occasionally ferrets with abscesses will develop septicaemia, so prompt treatment is always recommended.

Actinomycosis

Actinomyces is a gram positive filamentous organism, which may be found as a normal inhabitant of the mouth. Occasionally *Actinomyces spp.* cause signs in ferrets similar to lumpy jaw in cattle, which is caused by *A. bovis*. Trauma to the mucosa allows the organism to penetrate and invade the tissues of the head and neck, bone, tongue, pharynx, lymph nodes, or lungs. The animal may present acutely with a high fever and a diffuse, hard swelling of the

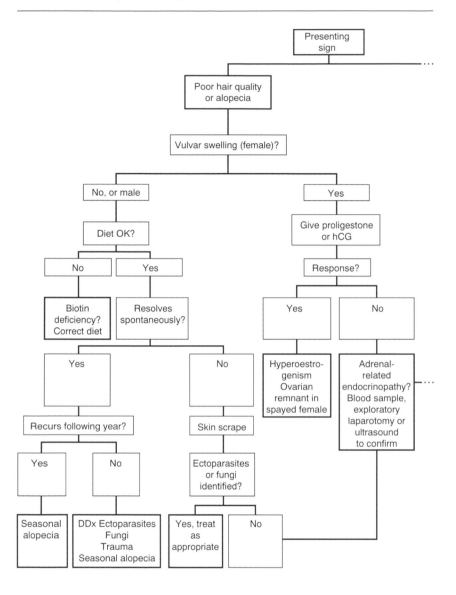

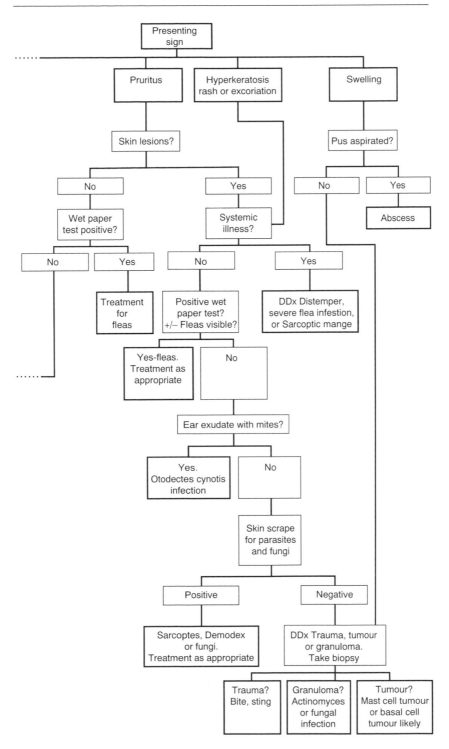

Figure 10.1 Diagnostic approach to skin lesions.

ventral neck, or the course may be more chronic, with cervical swellings and sinus tracts developing over days or weeks. The swelling may appear to be a tumour, so perform a biopsy. Characteristically the mass consists of a chronic pyogranuloma with 'sulphur granules', pockets of yellowish green material containing microcolonies and calcium phosphate crystals, within a fibrous mass. A resolution of the signs may be achieved by prolonged treatment with cephalosporins (e.g. Ceporex, Schering-Plough), or other antibiotic following sensitivity testing. In some cases it may be necessary to debride the affected tissues surgically to provide drainage. Liquid feeding is also beneficial, particularly where the tissues of the neck are swollen and eating solids is uncomfortable.

Ectoparasites

Ear mites

Otodectes cynotis, the ear mite commonly found in dogs and cats, is also common in ferrets, particularly young kits and old animals. The adult mite spends its entire life in the ears, rarely venturing onto the body, and spreads between animals by direct contact. Eggs are laid singly, and take three weeks to develop into adults. Often, there are no clinical signs, or there may be pruritus, leading to rubbing the ears or shaking the head. Occasionally there may be secondary bacterial infection which can lead to otitis media and a head tilt. On examination, there is inflammation of the ear canal with a thick, brown or black waxy exudate. Adult mites, larvae and eggs are easily visible in the exudate under a microscope.

Treat all susceptible animals in the household concurrently. First, clean the ears of the affected animals(s) using a proprietary cleaner (this will probably require general anaesthesia) before using an insecticide. Ivermectin (Panomec, Merial), at 200–400 µg/kg by subcutaneous injection can be curative, and appears to last long enough to kill the hatching eggs. It can be safely repeated after two weeks if required. Alternatively, a few drops of ivermectin or a permethrin based product such as GAC drops (Arnolds Veterinary

Products), which also contains local anaesthetic and antibiotic, can be massaged into the ear canal weekly.

Eradication of *Otodectes cynotis* from a ferret colony can be achieved by treatment of all individuals in the colony with ivermectin every three weeks for three or four treatments.

Fleas

Ferrets can become infested with *Ctenocephalides spp,* particularly between July and October, which may cause no clinical signs, or cause pruritus which may be intense. Sometimes there may be alopecia, and in heavy infestations there can be anaemia, which can be fatal. The infestation may be diagnosed by identifying the parasites in the animal's coat, or by brushing the animal over a piece of wet paper and looking for flea faeces which will turn red in contact with the water. Ferrets can usually be treated with products designed for cats: all susceptible animals in the household and the environment should be treated simultaneously. Collars are not recommended for use in ferrets. When using sprays, it is helpful to spray the product onto a cloth or glove, then rub that into the animal's fur.

Sarcoptic mange

Sarcoptic mange may be encountered occasionally. There is an intensely pruritic whole body form, or a more localised form which affects just the feet, which is sometimes called 'foot rot'. Affected animals may have generalised pruritus with crusting and excoriation, or swelling of the foot with self mutilation and loss of the nails. If untreated, the foot can be lost. Treat by trimming the nails, and soaking the feet to remove the scabs. Give ivermectin at $400\,\mu g/kg$ and repeat in two weeks: this will usually produce a resolution of signs with both forms of the disease, and can be repeated if required. Systemic antibiotics can be given to control secondary bacterial infection. Corticosteroids can be used with caution to control the pruritus, or shampoos can be used, e.g. 0.5% carbaryl, weekly for three to five weeks. Care should be taken with organophosphates in ferrets as safe levels have not been established. The environment should be thoroughly disinfected while treatment is taking place, or the animal transferred to a clean cage.

Other parasite infestations

Demodex may be encountered very rarely in immunosuppressed animals, causing hyperkeratosis. Diagnosis in such animals may be made by a deep skin scraping, which will reveal the presence of cigar shaped mites. Frequent treatment with amitraz can be curative.

Harvest mites can be found in small multiple lesions on the underside of the neck and trunk in August and September. The small orange mites can be seen in scrapings from the lesions.

Ticks are found on ferrets occasionally in spring and autumn. Working ferrets which regularly go down burrows can get heavy infestations with ticks. Remove these carefully, taking care to ensure the mouthparts are not left in the animal.

Myiasis may occur if wounds are invaded by dipterous larvae. Clean and irrigate the wound, then apply an insecticide, and give antibiotics as appropriate. Owners must be encouraged to pay closer attention to their ferrets if this occurs.

Other infectious causes

Fungal infections

Dermatomycosis (ringworm) is uncommon in ferrets. Young animals or older immunosuppressed animals may develop areas of crusty alopecia, with brittle hair and evidence of broken hair shafts. In immunosuppressed animals the infection can become generalised. *Microsporum canis* has been associated with transient infections in young kits, which usually resolve spontaneously. A diagnosis can be made by microscopic examination of skin and hair samples and fungal culture, or rarely *M. canis* will fluoresce under ultra-violet light. Ringworm can be treated by clipping the hair around the affected areas and applying iodine scrubs or keratolytic shampoos. Treatment with griseofulvin 25 mg/kg daily for three weeks is also effective, but should not be given to pregnant females. The environment should also be disinfected thoroughly to eliminate spores. *M. Canis* will usually be caught from an infected cat, so check in-contact cats and treat if necessary.

Fungal infections may also be suspected in animals which have persistent skin eruptions and draining tracts which are unresponsive to antibiotics. Such infections are usually accompanied by other signs such as pneumonia and chronic weight loss.

Malassezia and other moulds can be associated with cases of otitis externa which are resistant to treatment. There may be crusting and necrosis of the pinna which can spread to the face. If untreated, the pinna may have to be amputated. This can be treated with a combination of oral ketoconazole at 5–10 mg/kg twice daily, topical antifungals, antibiotics and prednisolone.

Canine distemper virus

Infection with this virus may cause hyperkeratosis of the footpads and a rash in the inguinal area and under the chin. Secondary bacterial pyoderma may also develop. Animals with distemper should be euthanased (see Chapter 6).

Non-infectious diseases

Alopecia

'Normal' alopecia

Alopecia or poor hair quality is a common presenting sign in ferrets, but is not always indicative of pathology. Often, it is a natural seasonal variation: the coat is frequently unkempt during the moults in spring and autumn, and may progress to alopecia. Both sexes may develop alopecia on the tail, perineum and inguinal area during the breeding season, and jills in particular can appear quite scruffy, the stress of gestation and lactation causing telogen effluvium. These cases of seasonal alopecia can recur the following year. Alopecia may occur just on the tail; the reason for this is unknown.

In all these cases, the hair regains its normal sleek appearance spontaneously within a few months.

Hormonal alopecia

Hormone imbalances such as hyperoestrogenism or adrenal-related endocrinopathy may lead to a typical endocrine alopecia. The hair loss is bilaterally symmetrical, beginning in areas of wear and tear such as the flanks, tail and inguinal region (see Plate 13). In cases of hyperoestrogenism, alopecia may be accompanied by petechiae or abrasions. These conditions are discussed in detail in Chapter 9, Endocrine Diseases.

Dietary alopecia

Dietary deficiencies may result in poor hair quality and a dull, dry coat. The inclusion of raw eggs can lead to biotin deficiency, since avidin in the egg white binds biotin, and has been reported to lead to alopecia.

Neoplasia

Neoplasms are fairly common in the skin of ferrets, and the incidence increases with age. In most cases, early excision will be curative. The commonest types are mast cell tumours and basal cell tumours (sebaceous cell epitheliomas), but other types of neoplasm which have been reported include sebaceous adenomas, squamous cell carcinoma, histiocytoma, haemangioma, and adenocarcinoma of the preputial or sweat glands. Mammary adenocarcinoma may also occur. These are rare and do not metastasise.

Mast cell tumours

These are commonly reported in the USA, but seem to be rare in the UK. They are found in both sexes, commonly on the neck, shoulders, or trunk. They appear as flat, raised, tan coloured or erythematous plaques up to 1 cm diameter, which may be pruritic, alopecic or hyperkeratotic. They can be covered with a black crusty exudate, and are often hidden under the hair. The diagnosis may be

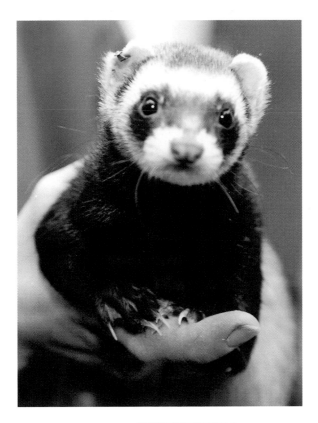

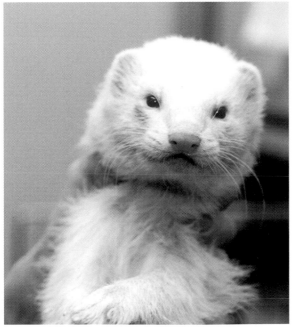

Varieties of the
ferret: **Plate 1**
(above) fitch,
sometimes called
polecat; **Plate 2**
(left) albino.

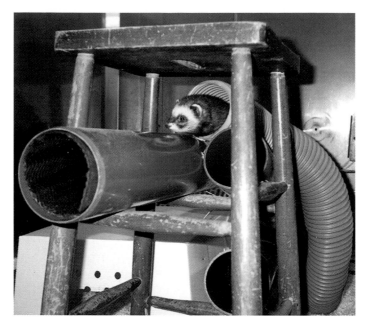

Plate 3 A young ferret enjoys playing in some artificial tunnels.

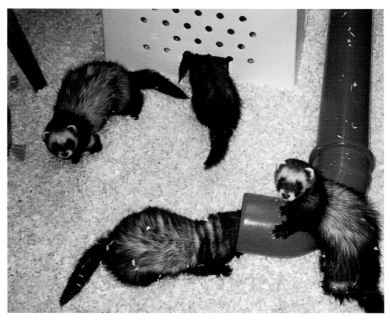

Plate 4 Group housed ferrets with lots of playthings.

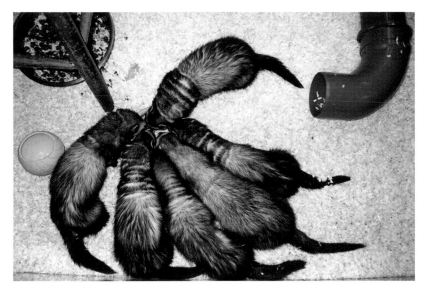

Plate 5 These group housed ferrets really enjoy their bowl of milk.

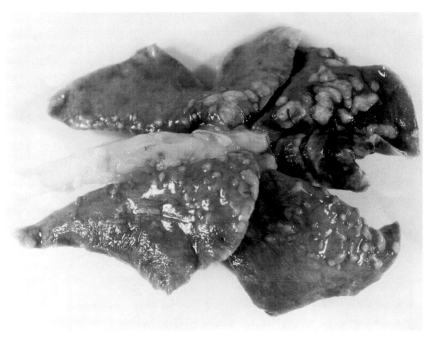

Plate 6 Endogenous lipid pneumonia, a common incidental finding at postmortem in ferrets.

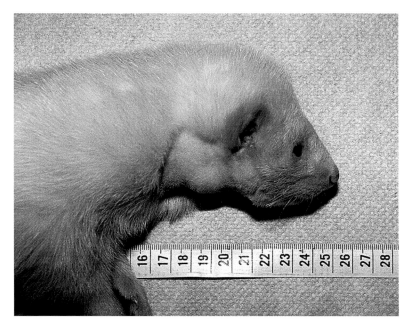

Plate 7 Salivary mucocoele at angle of jaw.

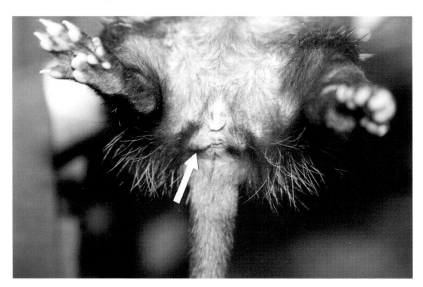

Plate 8 Impacted anal gland (arrow).

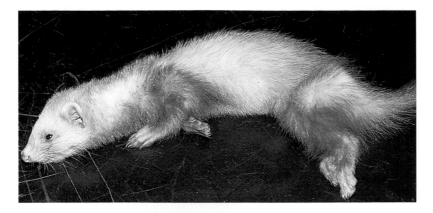

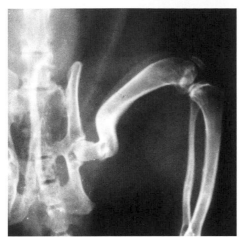

Plate 9 Ferret with posterior paresis.

Plate 10 Healed pathological fracture of the femur and deformities in tibia and fibula in an adult animal which had osteodystrophy as a juvenile.

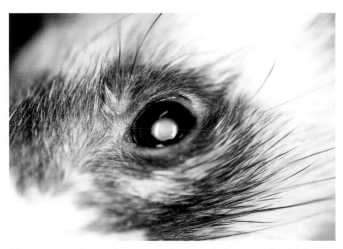

Plate 11 Unilateral cataract in an eight month old ferret. The lesion developed over a few days and led to total blindness in the affected eye.

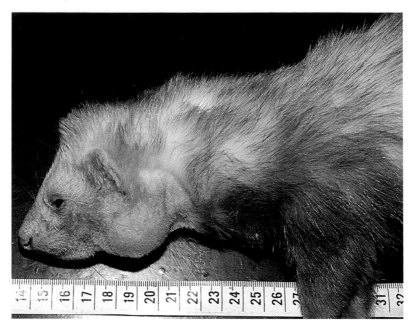

Plate 12 Submandibular abscess.

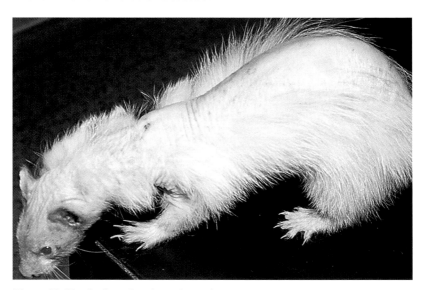

Plate 13 Typical endocrine alopecia.

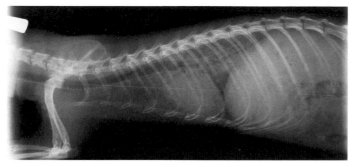

Plate 14 Note the enlarged, globoid shape of the heart, dorsal elevation of the trachea and diffuse lung pattern in this ferret with cardiomyopathy.

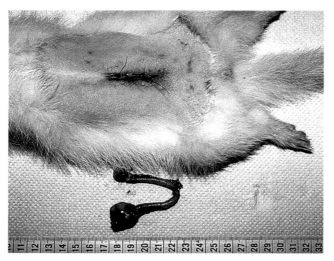

Plate 15 Ovarian thecoma in a jill.

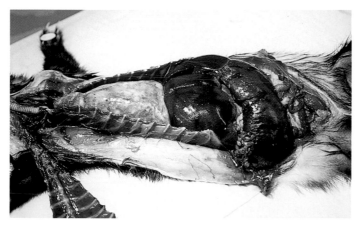

Plate 16 Postmortem examination of a juvenile ferret with lymphosarcoma. Note the massive splenic enlargement and the thymic mass causing compression of the lungs.

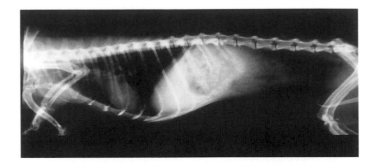

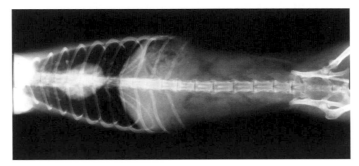

Normal radiographs: **Plate 17** (top) lateral; **Plate 18** (below) dorso-ventral.

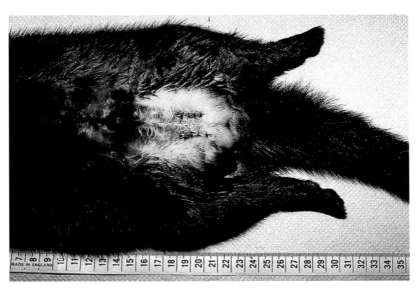

Plate 19 Site for vasectomy incisions (shown in a mink).

confirmed by taking a fine needle aspirate or an excisional biopsy. Usually, they are well differentiated and relatively benign, and may disappear and recur over time. Excision of the lesion is curative.

Basal cell tumours (sebaceous epithelioma)

These appear as warty lesions anywhere on the body, particularly the head and neck, and are common in females over five years of age. They can grow rapidly and may ulcerate. They consist of basal cells, some of which may show sebaceous or squamous differentiation. They are non-malignant and removal is usually successful.

Other non-infectious causes

Bites and stings

Insect stings or snake bites can occur in ferrets, and may present as erythematous painful or pruritic swellings, with or without evidence of puncture marks. Symptomatic treatment is sufficient for most insect stings, but anti-venom is recommended for bites from venomous snakes.

Iatrogenic alopecia

Small, well circumscribed patches of alopecia have been reported following subcutaneous injections of proligestone, if the site is not massaged sufficiently at the time of injection.

Allergies, contact dermatitis and other non-specific dermatoses have been reported in ferrets, but only rarely.

Self trauma

Ferrets kept in an inadequate environment with nowhere to hide may rub their faces as they try to find a bolt-hole, leading to abrasions and broken hairs.

11 REPRODUCTIVE, PERIPARTURIENT AND NEONATAL DISEASES

Breeding ferrets is by no means an easy task, and the management of a breeding colony must be very good if it is to be successful. A considerable amount of intensive care needs to be given to the jill and kits during gestation, parturition and lactation. Even in well managed colonies, 10% of kits may be lost before weaning, and losses will be much greater if nutrition and management are poor. The main single factor in determining the success or not of a breeding program is nutrition of the jill. Poor nutrition can lead to small litters, pregnancy toxaemia, or failure to conceive. More details of breeding can be found in Chapter 4.

DISEASES OF THE JILL

Pregnancy toxaemia

Aetiology and pathogenesis

This life threatening condition is seen in jills mainly in late gestation, although it can occur at other times. The aetiology is believed to be similar to that in guinea pigs, where a negative energy balance in late gestation combined with stress leads to the breakdown of fats to provide energy. The result is hepatic lipidosis and ketosis, which cause clinical signs. Typically, it affects primiparous jills carrying an average litter and being fed an average or poor quality diet which experience a period of anorexia in late gestation, whether due to transport, change of diet or other reason. It may also occur in jills carrying large litters on good quality diets. It can occur after a period of anorexia as short as 24 hours.

Clinical signs

The jill develops sudden lethargy and weakness in late pregnancy, and can become dehydrated, with black, tarry stools. There may be hypothermia, and can be some loss of hair. The jill will be hypoglycaemic, and ketones may be detectable in blood or urine. Death may occur acutely with few clinical signs. At post mortem examination, the liver is pale and fatty, there may be a degree of anaemia and some gastric ulceration.

Diagnosis

These clinical signs in a jill in late gestation are highly suggestive of pregnancy toxaemia.

Treatment and control

It is important to remove the source of the stress as soon as possible, so a caesarean section should be performed at once. If the caesarean is carried out before 40 days of gestation, the kits are unlikely to survive. It may be possible in some cases to stabilise the jill and nourish her until it is safe to deliver the kits if her condition is not too bad. However, the prognosis is poor even with prompt treatment, and success depends upon the degree of hepatic infiltration. Induce anaesthesia using an inhalation agent, since the jill may not be able to metabolise injectable agents effectively, and give an infusion of glucose intravenously throughout the procedure. Provide extra heating to counteract any hypothermia. Post operatively, take care to maintain the animal's hydration status, and offer her frequent, small, high calorie meals. The jill will need intensive treatment including fluids and supplementary heating until she is eating adequate quantities.

The condition can be prevented by ensuring the jill is eating a good quality diet and drinking sufficiently throughout gestation. Make sure more than one source of water is provided, for example give a bottle and a bowl, and put several food bowls down so if one spills she will still have access to another. High calorie nutritional supplements may also be given e.g. Nutri-plus gel, Virbac.

Pseudopregnancy

This may occur if implantation fails or if the mating is unsuccessful, which can occur if an immature male is used for breeding or if there is insufficient light in the month before breeding. A period of pseudopregnancy also follows treatment with hCG for prolonged oestrus or mating with a vasectomised male. Pseudopregnancy typically lasts 41–43 days, the vulval swelling recedes, the jill's abdomen swells and she may have mammary development and exhibit nest building behaviour. No treatment is required.

Dystocia

Dystocia is fairly common in ferrets, with an incidence of approximately 1%. There are several causes, including large kits (see below), malpresentation, deformed or anasarcous fetuses. Under normal conditions, a jill will litter over a period of two to three hours. If she has been straining for considerably longer than this medical intervention or a caesarean may be indicated. Occasionally, the jill may give birth to one or more kits then appear to cease parturition, even when more kits are palpable. In these cases there may be uterine inertia, and doses of oxytocin (0.2–3.0 units/kg, by i.m injection) and/or calcium borogluconate may be beneficial. Care must be taken to ensure the cervix is open when using oxytocin, as in other species. If there is no response to oxytocin, perform a caesarean.

A condition similar to 'single pup syndrome' in dogs exists in ferrets where if there are only one or two kits, the hormonal stimulus to initiate parturition seems to be insufficient. Gestation normally lasts 41–42 days. Beyond this, the kits in a small litter may grow too large to be able to pass through the birth canal (above about 15 g), and dystocia and death of the kits are common in these cases. If it appears that there is a small litter, induce parturition on day 41 of gestation. Give the jill 0.5 mg prostaglandin $F_2\alpha$ (Lutalyse, Pharmacia and Upjohn) by i.m. injection, and follow it one to four hours later with 6 units oxytocin i.m. This will induce parturition within two to twelve hours in most cases. If treatment is not successful within eight hours, it can be repeated or a caesarean performed.

Poor litter size

Primiparous jills usually have around eight kits, subsequent litters are larger. Many factors may be involved if litters are small. Mating with a hob of low fertility, mating only once or at the wrong time during the breeding season, or breeding animals which carry lethal recessive genes can be involved, but poor nutrition is the most common factor. Poor reproductive performance may also be seen in jills with Aleutian disease virus infection in the absence of any other signs.

Animals destined for breeding should be fed a high quality diet from weaning, with 35 to 40% animal protein, and 18 to 20% fat. If she is finicky during gestation, offer the jill a variety of premium foods: she is unlikely to reject all of them. See Chapter 3 for more details of ferret nutrition.

Poor mothering

Primiparous jills may take several days to begin nursing, by which time many kits have died. They may appear to be frightened of their kits, and the problem is exacerbated if the jill is disturbed shortly after parturition or if there are fluctuations in temperature. Handling the kits is not necessarily a problem, but if combined with excess noise or other disturbances then problems are likely. The jill may simply reject the kits, bury them in litter, or even cannibalise them. To prevent this, the jill should be allowed to litter down in a quiet place in a well ventilated nest box with the ambient temperature no more than 21°C to avoid heat stroke.

Normally, the nest box should contain the kits but allow the jill to get out. If a primiparous jill has rejected but not cannibalised her kits, try confining her with the kits in a well ventilated cage until she has begun nursing, only allowing her out to feed. Alternatively, the jill may be distracted by giving her a favourite food or treat and holding her gently in place while the babies suck. Usually, the jill will settle down after a few days.

Occasionally, the jill will allow the babies to start sucking but will pull away abruptly. This may be due to pain or discomfort, and may be resolved by the application of a small amount of emollient or corticosteroid cream to the nipples, allowing this to remain in place for several minutes before washing it off and allowing the kits to suck.

Lactation failure

Shortly after birth, the kits seek a nipple and start to suck. Some jills will allow kits to nurse as soon as they are born, in between the births of subsequent kits, and others wait until parturition is over and suckle all kits at once. Once the whole litter is nursing, the milk supply is usually established very rapidly. However, sometimes lactation fails despite the attempts of the kits to suck. In these cases, the kits will cry continually and keep trying to nurse, and if this is not spotted quickly, the kits will die.

There are many common causes of lactation failure, which are discussed below. If all these have been ruled out, the jill may have an underlying genetic incapability of producing milk, and using her for breeding in the future should be discouraged. Fostering or hand rearing (see Chapter 4) will be necessary in these cases. Fostering kits is relatively easy, provided the kits are warm and active. If not, warm them up and administer a little glucose solution to revive the kits before fostering them.

Management

If a jill is poorly managed, particularly a primiparous jill, she may never settle down with her kits and her milk supply will dry up. She should be left undisturbed in a quiet place which is not too hot, with easy access to food and water until she has bonded with the kits and is nursing them adequately. If the jill has had a prolonged or difficult labour, she may be exhausted and offering her some palatable high calorie supplement and fluids during and after birth may be all that is needed. Occasionally the jill will be uncomfortable and may need some analgesic, such as flunixin (Finadyne, Schering Plough) – give her 0.1 ml. The milk let down reflex can be elicited by the admin-istration of a small dose of oxytocin, given i.m. Giving the kits a few drops of glucose syrup will give them an extra impetus to find the nipple and begin sucking, and once they are sucking strongly, the milk supply will probably become established quickly.

Small litters

Lactation failure can occur with litters smaller than five, since this appears to be the critical number of kits required to maintain lactation. The litter can be fostered relatively easily onto another jill, or surplus kits from another litter can be added to make a large enough litter to maintain lactation.

Nutrition

Nutrition of the jill has a profound effect on the quality of lactation. A jill on a maintenance diet will produce poor milk and have slow growing kits with poor coats. She should be given a premium diet in lactation, reaching a fat level of 30% by two to three weeks post partum. The kits can be supplemented with moist food and milk replacer, but a good supply of ferret milk is best. Dehydration can also have adverse effects on the milk supply, so plenty of fresh water must always be available.

Systemic disease

If the jill is unwell for any reason, her milk supply will drop. The kits will be thin and crying and will tend to crawl around rather than staying with the jill. Commonly, this will be associated with mastitis or metritis, which are covered in more detail below. If systemic infections are treated promptly, the jill will continue lactating and generally the kits should be left with her so she may continue to feed them as soon as she is able, although jills infected early in lactation may experience a complete failure of the milk supply. Supplement the kits with milk replacer (see page 99) four times daily during the period the jill is ill, and ensure she has excellent nutrition, enhancing her diet with high calorie supplements if required.

Acute mastitis

Aetiology and pathogenesis

Acute mastitis is quite common in ferrets, and occurs either immediately after parturition, or at peak lactation when the kits are three weeks old and place great demands on the jill. Causative agents commonly isolated include staphylococci and coliforms, and these probably enter the gland through minute breaks in the skin, possibly caused by sucking kits. Coliform mastitis is particularly common if there is faecal contamination of the environment. Mastitis can take the form of cellulitis, mammary abscessation, or necrotic mastitis. If untreated, the infection may become systemic. The mouths of sucking kits can act as sources of infection for adjacent glands and other jills acting as foster mothers.

Clinical signs

Clinically, one or more mammary glands will be swollen, red and painful, with congestion, oedema and sometimes haemorrhages affecting the glands and surrounding tissues. The jill can be anorexic, lethargic and reluctant to nurse, and may develop systemic signs including pyrexia, nasal discharge, and diarrhoea. Staphylococcal infections are suppurative, and the lactiferous ducts become distended with pus and inflammatory oedema. Mammary abscesses are large, fluctuant swellings which will eventually burst, exuding copious purulent material. In cases of necrotic mastitis due to *E. coli*, large areas of diffuse, severe coagulative and liquefactive necrosis develop which extend into adjacent tissues. The affected area can become gangrenous within hours of infection: the tissues turn black with clear demarcation of infarcted areas, and the jill becomes very ill and dehydrated due to endotoxaemia. Such cases are life threatening and need prompt treatment.

Diagnosis

The clinical signs are diagnostic. Often, the milk appears normal, although bacteria may be present, and culture and sensitivity should be performed routinely.

Treatment and control

In most cases, leave the kits with their mother, rather than fostering them to another jill. There are several reasons for this. The kits are likely to have been the source of the infection, so fostering them may simply spread the disease to the foster mother. In addition, if the kits are removed, the jill's milk supply will dry up and she will not be able to feed them when she recovers. Emptying the infected gland of milk is a common treatment for mastitis in other species, and leaving the kits with the jill is the easiest way to achieve this in ferrets. The kits may need to be supplemented with milk replacer (see page 99) while the jill is recovering, but they should be left with her. If the jill is treated rapidly, she will continue to nurse them.

Treat straightforward cases of mastitis as follows. Strict hygiene is important to avoid spreading the infection to other jills, so hands must be washed carefully after handling an affected jill and litter. Give antibiotics according to culture and sensitivity, and give the jill extra fluids, vitamins and nutritional supplements. Apply hot compresses frequently to the affected glands, to ease any discomfort and 'draw out' the infection. Turn the jill at regular intervals so the kits are encouraged to rotate and use different nipples, and encourage the strongest kits to suck from the affected glands to empty them. To prevent enteritis in the kits, give them a few drops of the same antibiotic the jill is receiving.

Treat mammary abscesses as in any other area, by providing drainage, and flushing the abscess cavity twice daily with dilute antiseptic solution.

Immediate aggressive therapy is required in cases of necrotic mastitis if the jill is to be saved. Remove the necrotic tissue using a scalpel: often no anaesthesia is required for this as the tissue is insensitive, or resect the area under general anaesthesia and suture using subcuticular sutures after insertion of a surgical drain. Give intravenous fluids and broad spectrum antibiotics, such as clavulanate potentiated amoxycillin (Synulox palatable drops, Pfizer, 0.25 ml/kg twice daily), preferably after culture and sensitivity. The condition is painful and may prevent the jill from nursing, so give her flunixin (Finadyne injection, Schering Plough, 2.5 mg twice daily) which will also counter any toxaemia. Following treatment, the jill may lose one or more glands, may experience recurrent mastitis, or may heal completely.

Mastitis is largely preventable by ensuring strict hygiene. The bedding (or litter, if used) in the latrine area should be changed once or twice daily, and the cage and litter box cleaned with disinfectant. The nest box should be sterilised when the bedding is changed, once or twice weekly. However, some cases will still occur. The causative agents are normal inhabitants of the gut, and when the kits begin to defaecate spontaneously at about three weeks of age there will be faecal matter in the nest box continually. Minor cases can be prevented from becoming serious by examining the jill daily, paying particular attention during the period between three and five weeks post partum. If there are any signs of redness or swelling in the mammary glands, give the jill a preventative five day course of a broad spectrum antibiotic such as amoxycillin.

Chronic mastitis

This disease usually appears insidiously when the kits are about three weeks old. The mammary glands become infected by bacteria, commonly *Staphylococcus intermedius,* and damaged tissues are gradually replaced by fibrous scar tissue, becoming firm although non-painful. Milk production falls, and the kits stop gaining weight although they may continue to grow in stature. The condition is very contagious, and affected jills should be kept away from other breeding jills. There is no effective treatment for affected jills – they will never be able to nurse again and euthanasia may be the only option for such a jill in a breeding colony. The kits of affected jills should be given vitamin supplementation, oral antibiotics and milk replacer. It is possible to foster them if care is taken not to transmit the infection. Leaving the kits away from both dams for a few hours should ensure their guts are empty of infected milk, then the kits can be carefully bathed using warm water or mild shampoo before being given to the foster mother.

Metritis and pyometra

Aetiology and pathogenesis

Metritis (inflammation of the uterus) and pyometra (accumulation of pus in the uterus) are uncommon but can occur during pseudo-pregnancy, typically three weeks after a failed mating or mating with a vasectomised male. There is cystic hyperplasia of the endometrium, followed by infection with organisms such as *E. coli,* staphylococci, streptococci or *Corynebacterium* spp. This can also occur secondary to hyperoestrogenism or other causes of immunosuppression.

Clinical signs

With metritis, the jill is depressed, lethargic, and pyrexic, and may have a vaginal discharge. Pyometra is characterised by a sudden onset of anorexia and depression with or without vaginal discharge, and the jill becomes very ill and toxaemic. Torsion of the infected uterine horns may occur.

Diagnosis

The signs are typical, and the enlarged uterus may be palpable or visible on x-ray.

Treatment

For metritis and cases of secondary infection, give antibiotics following culture and sensitivity and treat the primary cause. Treatment for hyperoestrogenism is discussed in Chapter 9, Endocrine Diseases. If the uterus is enlarged and the cervix is closed, the administration of 0.5 mg prostaglandin $F_2\alpha$ (Lutalyse, Pharmacia and Upjohn) followed by antibiotic treatment can be successful. In cases of pyometra, the toxaemia can be life threatening and rapid treatment is needed. Give the animal fluid therapy, and remove the infected uterus under general anaesthesia, preferably using isoflurane.

Perivulvar dermatitis and vaginitis

A copious mucoserous discharge is produced during oestrus which can cause the perineum, hindlegs and inguinal areas to become very wet, predisposing to perivulvar dermatitis and infection. In addition, the enlarged vulva may be abraded or irritated by bedding material, and can become infected and sore. Clinically the vulva is moist, and ulceration or erosion of the perivulvar skin or vaginal mucosa may be visible. Remove the cause of the irritation and place the animal onto more suitable bedding such as artificial sheepskin. Cleanse the affected area with a suitable antiseptic such as chlorhexidine, dry thoroughly and apply a barrier cream to protect the skin in the inguinal region. Applying emollient or debriding creams such as Dermisol (Pfizer) to the vulva can also be beneficial, and systemic antibiotics may be needed in severe cases.

Hypocalcaemia (milk fever)

This occurs occasionally at peak lactation, three to four weeks post partum. The jill may present with posterior paralysis, hyperaesthesia or convulsions. Diagnosis may be made on the history and clinical signs. Treatment with calcium borogluconate by intraperitoneal injection is usually successful. Dose to effect, starting with 1–2 mls. The condition can be prevented by adding a balanced vitamin and mineral supplement to the diet of lactating jills.

DISEASES OF THE NEONATAL KIT

Mortality in ferret kits can be high. The kits are born with no hair, weighing 6–12 g, and have difficulty maintaining their body temperature for the first two weeks. They should weigh 30 g at one week, 60–70 g by two weeks, and 100 g by three weeks. Healthy kits should lie quietly by their mother, either nursing or sleeping. They begin to explore and nibble soft foods from three weeks of age. If the kits are healthy but the jill cannot rear them at all, hand rearing is difficult, particularly for kits less than one week old. Most nursing jills will accept extra kits at any age and fostering is easy. The best solution in most cases is to supplement the kits but leave them with their mother, so the stimulus to produce milk remains and the jill can provide warmth and stimulate urination and defaecation etc. Puppy or kitten milk replacer can be used, mixed with cream to raise the fat content to approximately 20% (three parts milk replacer to one part cream). Feed the warm milk individually to the kits from a dropper bottle, three or four times daily, giving as much as the kit will take. After four weeks, the kits may begin drinking from a dish. A low, flat dish with a rim is best, since ferrets like to put their feet on the edge of the dish while drinking and this will cause a saucer to tip over. At about this time, the kits will begin to take solid food, and from five weeks they can be given adult food and will survive without milk if required.

Kits are particularly prone to dehydration, hypothermia and hypoglycaemia, and deaths within the first three days of birth are usually due to malformations, being cannibalised by the jill, becoming entangled with the placenta, failure to nurse, or maternal neglect.

Hypothermia

If the jill is ill or a poor mother, the kits will become cold and will not nurse. They can be revived by giving them a few drops of glucose by mouth, then warming them up slowly in the hand or with a heating pad. Warmed fluids can be given by subcutaneous injection. They can then be replaced with the jill or fostered as necessary.

Entangled umbilical cords, infection and septicaemia

Occasionally, the umbilical cords and placentae of littermates become entangled, particularly if the litter is large and labour is rapid so the jill cannot chew off the placentae. The kits cannot nurse and rapidly become hypothermic and hypoglycaemic. The jill may try to separate them later and in the process cause more trauma and prolapse of the umbilical cords. If this occurs, soften the placentae with warm water, remove any pieces of sawdust or bedding stuck to the mass, and cut the umbilical cords individually as far from the kits as possible. To prevent this from occurring, supervise births from a distance, and trim any long umbilical cords or placentae which remain attached.

In any case, ascending infections from the umbilical stumps can occur if hygiene is poor and the stumps are not disinfected soon after birth, particularly if the jill has a concurrent infection. This causes the kits to become distressed and dehydrated, hypothermic, bloated and anorexic. Warmth, fluids and antibiotics can be given to the kits, but the prognosis is guarded.

Other causes of infection in the neonate

Diarrhoea

Rotavirus, *E. coli* and *Campylobacter* may all cause disease in neonatal kits. Again, maternal infections such as mastitis may be a predisposing factor. Rotavirus may be carried in the adult ferret, affecting kits which have not acquired passive immunity. In kits up to one week old, it causes diarrhoea and dehydration. They may appear wet with a sticky coat, although the jill may clean them so no signs are apparent. The kits can die from dehydration, so fluids should be given orally or by subcutaneous injection. Oral antibiotic drops may prevent any secondary infections.

Diseases in the kits will cause them to be anorexic, so it is important to check the jill as well, since if the kits are not nursing she may develop mastitis or agalactia.

Ophthalmia neonatorum

This can occur in kits from a few days to three weeks old, before the eyes open. A purulent exudate from the conjunctiva causes the lids to swell. Drainage should be established, and can be achieved using a scalpel or needle to open the lids along the suture line. Clean the exudate away carefully twice daily, and apply antibiotic ointment, such as cloxacillin (Orbenin, Pfizer). The condition is contagious so all littermates should be checked daily.

12 CARDIOVASCULAR DISEASES

APPROACH TO CARDIOVASCULAR DISEASES

There have been few published studies of cardiovascular disease in ferrets, although cardiac problems appear to be increasingly diagnosed in middle aged to older ferrets.

Clinical signs

The signs of cardiac disease are often vague and non-specific, and include lethargy, weight loss and inappetence. Hind leg weakness is common, and there may be tachypnoea, hypothermia, or abdominal enlargement (due to ascites). The 'cardiac cough' is rare in ferrets. Cardiac disease may be discovered as an incidental finding on clinical examination, and if the animal is compensating well there may be no clinical signs at all.

Clinical examination may reveal cyanosis with a prolonged capillary refill time, jugular distension or pulsation, and pulse deficits or a weak, thready pulse. Auscultation of the heart should be done between the sixth and eighth ribs, which is more caudal to the position of the heart in the cat. A pronounced sinus arrhythmia is common. Features observed in cases of cardiac disease may include left or right sided holosystolic murmur, tachycardia, gallop rhythm, muffling of heart sounds or pulmonary crackles. It is common for there to be tachypnoea, dyspnoea or both, associated with pulmonary oedema, and there may be hepatosplenomegaly or ascites.

Diagnosis

The diagnosis of cardiovascular disease can be made on the history and clinical examination, and confirmed by radiography, electrocardiography and ultrasound examination. It may also be necessary to perform haematology and biochemistry, or examination of fluid removed by thoracocentesis or abdominocentesis, since cardiac disease in older ferrets is often accompanied by other systemic diseases.

Changes found on radiography include a globoid cardiac silhouette, pleural effusion, and a diffuse interstitial pattern associated with pulmonary oedema (see Plate 14). There may also be hepatosplenomegaly and ascites.

Electrocardiography is important for the diagnosis of arrhythmias and conduction disorders, and any changes need to be correlated with other data before interpretation. It is best to record the ECG in the unsedated animal if possible, but if necessary the recording can be carried out using isoflurane/oxygen anaesthesia. For a full description of the ECG in ferrets see Bone *et al.* (1988) and Smith and Bishop (1985). Briefly, the ECG in ferrets differs from that in the dog and the cat in that the lead II P-waves are small, but the R-waves are large. The QT interval is short, and elevation of the ST segment is common. Changes seen commonly in cardiac disease include sinus tachycardia, and atrial or ventricular premature contractions. Bradycardia and conduction disturbances are rarely associated with primary cardiac disease, but are usually secondary to extensive generalised disease and carry a grave prognosis.

Ultrasound is a useful tool in the diagnosis and evaluation of cardiac disease. This can be performed in the conscious animal held in lateral recumbency by the scruff of the neck and around the hips. It is possible to examine the size, shape, and function of the chambers of the heart, check for any pleural or pericardial effusion, and investigate any masses within the heart or anterior mediastinum. A common clinical finding is mild aortic valve insufficiency, but this is rarely associated with clinical signs and its significance is unknown.

Treatments for cardiac disease

Treatment regimes for cardiac disease in ferrets are often extrapolated from those used in cats and dogs. There will often be other
diseases present, so any treatment must be given carefully in the
light of this. It is often best to give supportive, non-specific therapies
initially, such as oxygen, diuretics, exercise restriction and low salt
diets, since the evaluation of cardiac function can be facilitated by
these treatments. Then, treatment with more specific drugs can be
given as necessary.

Treatments which have been used in the treatment of cardiac
disease in ferrets include:

- Frusemide (Lasix, Hoechst): 1–4 mg/kg two or three times daily,
  p.o., i.v., i.m., or s.c.
- Thiazide diuretics: use feline doses
- Adrenergic blockers, e.g. propanolol: 2–5 mg/kg once daily or in
  divided doses for the control of tachydysrhythmias
- Digoxin: 0.01 mg/kg p.o. once daily, increasing to twice daily
  according to clinical signs. Calculate the dose based on the lean
  body weight – generally it may be assumed that fat comprises
  15% of body weight, but there will need to be adjustment due to
  the seasonal fluctuation in body fat levels. Check closely for side
  effects such as vomiting or diarrhoea, inappetence, or arrhythmias, and do not use if the animal has azotaemia, hypokalaemia
  or frequent ventricular arrhythmias
- Vasodilators: Ferrets are quite sensitive to the effects of vasodilators and may become hypotensive and lethargic, but they can be
  used with caution. ACE inhibitors are balanced vasodilators,
  reducing both preload and afterload and helping to maintain
  cardiac output while reducing oedema. Enalapril (Cardiovet,
  Intervet) can be used at 0.5 mg/kg p.o. every 48 hours. Increase
  the dose slowly to 0.5 mg/kg once daily as required if there are no
  side effects. Nitroglycerin acts just as a venous dilator, reducing
  preload. Use 3–4 mm Nitroglycerin 2% ointment applied to the
  skin once or twice daily to help reduce pulmonary oedema.

DISEASES

Dilated/congestive cardiomyopathy

Aetiology and pathogenesis

This is probably the most common cardiac disorder in the ferret, and is increasingly recognised in middle aged to older animals. The aetiology is unknown, but it may sometimes be secondary to viral infections.

Clinical signs

Affected animals develop lethargy, weight loss, anorexia, depression, exercise intolerance and respiratory distress over a period of several months. On clinical examination, there may be cyanosis of the mucous membranes, hypothermia, muffled heart and lung sounds with moist rales and crackles, tachycardia with a systolic murmur, ascites and hind leg weakness. Radiography will show an enlarged globoid heart with increased sternal contact, dorsal elevation of the trachea, diffuse lung densities or pleural fluid, and may show ascites, or hepatosplenomegaly (see plate 14). The ECG will show many changes, including premature contractions, tall wide QRS complexes, increased R-wave amplitude associated with ventricular enlargement, and ST segment depression. Ultrasound examination will show enlargement of all four heart chambers, with reduced fractional shortening and possibly mitral and tricuspid regurgitation.

Post mortem examination will show dilatation of all four heart chambers, and occasionally areas of myocardial fibrosis may be grossly visible. In severe cases, there will be fluid in the pericardium, pleural cavity and abdominal cavity, which may cause focal collapse of the lungs. Sometimes the liver and spleen are large, firm and dark red due to chronic congestion.

Diagnosis

The diagnosis can be made on the clinical signs and radiography, and confirmed by ultrasonography.

Treatment and control

Treatment is aimed at maintaining cardiac output by manipulating the heart rate and rhythm, increasing contractility and reducing preload and afterload. If the animal presents acutely with profound dyspnoea, give oxygen, diuretics and perform thoracocentesis immediately. Once the animal has stabilised, begin treatment with vasodilators and digoxin. A low salt diet and exercise restriction can be of benefit. Taurine has been used with success in cases of cardiomyopathy in cats, and 250 mg p.o. once daily may produce a clinical improvement in ferrets also, although there is no data to support this (see Moneva-Jordan, 1998).

The response to treatment can be monitored by improvements in clinical signs, and by radiography and ultrasound. The prognosis in cases of dilated cardiomyopathy varies from poor to good: cases which are caught early may be expected to survive for up to 12 months post diagnosis, whereas others which present later may progress rapidly and require euthanasia within a few weeks or months. Treatment failure is not uncommon.

Hypertrophic cardiomyopathy

This is rare in ferrets. Hyperthyroidism is not reported in the ferret, so the common aetiology seen in cats is not recognised. Clinically there may be no signs, a left sided systolic murmur, or sudden death. The condition may best be diagnosed using ultrasound, to demonstrate thickening of the left ventricular free wall and interventricular septum. Treatment is aimed at reducing congestion with diuretics, and improving diastolic function. Heart rate can be reduced by using β-blockers such as propanolol, or calcium channel blockers. These improve diastolic filling and relax the myocardium.

Valvular heart disease

Valvular insufficiency affects mainly middle aged animals. There is thickening and myxomatous degeneration of the heart valves with atrial enlargement similar to that seen in dogs. Clinically there may be a holosystolic murmur, usually over the left apical region, and there may be moist lung sounds also. Diagnosis may be made on clinical signs and ultrasound. Treatment with diuretics and ACE inhibitors will reduce congestion. Digoxin may be indicated in the presence of supraventricular arrhythmias or if there is impairment of systolic function.

Myocarditis

Infections of the myocardium can occur in many diseases, including Aleutian disease, toxoplasmosis, or bacterial sepsis. The signs will vary depending on the organism and the extent of myocardial involvement. Ventricular arrhythmias with no cardiac enlargement are suspicious of myocarditis.

Heartworm disease

Dirofilaria immitis infection can occur in animals imported from areas where the disease exists. The parasite is transmitted by and undergoes development in a mosquito, and the disease is found where the parasite, mosquito and susceptible hosts coexist. In the UK, it will only be seen in animals imported from areas where it is endemic, e.g. Florida, Japan and Australia. The adult worms are found in the anterior vena cava, right ventricle or pulmonary artery, where they cause signs of right sided congestive heart failure. Due to the small size of the ferret heart, even a single worm can result in clinical signs. Often, the signs are vague, and include lethargy, coughing, dyspnoea, and ascites. Diagnosis can be difficult, since the microfilariae are not always present in peripheral blood, and tests for heartworm antigens are not always accurate. Consider this as a differential diagnosis if similar signs occur in imported animals. Treat affected animals with anthelminthics and anticoagulants, which reduce the risk of pulmonary emboli. Treatment with thiacetarsamide should be combined with heparin (100 i.u. given s.c. once daily for 21 days), then aspirin 22 mg/kg p.o. once daily for three months. The prognosis is poor and animals often succumb within one month of presentation. Give preventive treatment with ivermectin 0.1 mg/kg s.c. to animals living in areas where the infection is endemic.

Other diseases affecting the cardiovascular system

Aleutian disease

Infection with this virus leads to hypergammaglobulinaemia and immune complex formation. Deposition of the immune complexes leads to glomerulonephritis and vasculitis. Haemorrhages from affected arterioles can lead to anaemia and pallor. This disease is covered in more detail in Chapter 8, Musculoskeletal and Neurologic Diseases. Diagnosis is made by counter-immunoelectrophoresis, and there is no specific treatment.

Splenomegaly and hypersplenism

An enlarged spleen is a common incidental finding in ferrets. Usually in these cases there is some mild extramedullary haemopoiesis or congestion, but rarely evidence of pathology such as splenic lymphoma may be found. Perform a thorough clinical examination in animals with splenomegaly, since it is often found in association with other unrelated diseases, such as Aleutian disease or sepsis. Always evaluate the size of the spleen by gentle palpation in the conscious animal, since many anaesthetics cause gross enlargement of the spleen and could lead to a misdiagnosis. Take care during palpation however as a friable spleen may easily rupture. Examination of the spleen using ultrasound may be useful, and fine needle aspirates can be taken if necessary. In a normal healthy animal with no other signs of disease, it is likely to be an insignificant finding, and no treatment is indicated. If some other primary disease is found, treatment may be given as appropriate. Splenectomy is indicated for conditions such as neoplasia, torsion or rupture. Occasionally, a grossly enlarged spleen can cause discomfort, leading to lethargy.

Splenectomy may be curative in these cases but should only be carried out if there is no other underlying cause for the problem.

Hypersplenism occurs if the spleen destroys one or more blood cell types to excess, leading to anaemia, leucopenia etc depending on the cell types destroyed. This is an extremely rare condition. The spleen may or may not be enlarged, and there will be abnormalities on haematology and hypercellularity of the bone marrow. Remove the spleen and give blood transfusions and treatment for secondary infections as required.

Anaemia

Anaemia is a relatively common finding in ferrets. As in other species, it may be due to an increased loss of red cells, which will lead to a marrow response, or decreased production, which will not lead to a marrow response. In either case, the signs may be vague and non-specific, such as lethargy, weakness and inappetence, or there may be more specific signs such as pallor, melaena, petechiae or ecchymoses, or frank haemorrhage. Diagnosis can be made on the history and clinical signs, haematology, and bone marrow biopsy, and treatment given according to the aetiology.

The most common cause of anaemia with a marrow response is haemorrhage, which may be due to a gastrointestinal foreign body or gastric ulcer, Aleutian disease, platelet deficiency, trauma or heavy flea infestation. Haemolytic anaemia has not been reported but could occur.

Anaemia due to decreased red cell production is most commonly associated with hyperoestrogenism, but can also occur with any chronic disease, with nutritional deficiencies or if there is bone marrow neoplasia.

References

Bone, L., Battles, A.H., Goldfarb, R.D. *et al.* (1988) Electrocardiographic values from clinically normal, anaesthetised ferrets (*Mustela putorius furo*). *American Journal of Veterinary Research*, **49**, pp. 1884–7.

Moneva-Jordan, A. (1998) What is your diagnosis? *Journal of Small Animal Practice*, **39**, pp. 263; 303.

Smith, S.H. and Bishop, S.P. (1985) The electrocardiogram of normal ferrets and ferrets with right ventricular hypertrophy. *Laboratory Animal Science*, **35**, pp. 268–71.

13 UROGENITAL DISEASES

Renal disease is uncommon in ferrets, although a number of conditions have been reported including chronic interstitial nephritis, glomerulonephritis and pyelonephritis (see below). Clinical signs which may be seen include depression, lethargy, inappetence and weight loss, polydipsia and polyuria, dehydration and pallor. If renal disease is suspected, palpate the kidneys for size and shape, and perform urinalysis, radiography and abdominal ultrasound. Serum biochemistry may show a rise in blood urea nitrogen, although in contrast with other species this may not be paralleled by a rise in creatinine. In advanced cases, there may be a non-regenerative anaemia. The cause of renal disease may be apparent following these tests, or a biopsy may be required. Treatment should be given for the primary cause of disease.

Urolithiasis

Aetiology and pathogenesis

Calculi in the bladder or kidneys of ferrets are occasionally seen, mainly in males but also in pregnant jills, particularly if fed a diet consisting of plant proteins. Cystic calculi are more common than renal calculi, and stones vary in size from multiple tiny grains to single large stones. The precise aetiology is unknown, but stone formation can occur secondarily to urinary tract infections or may depend on the mineral component and protein level in the diet. The commonest crystal type is magnesium ammonium phosphate (struvite). Diets which are high in animal protein result in more acidic urine (pH 6) and struvite crystal formation is inhibited in such an environment. One report documented uroliths in 14% of a population of ferrets fed a commercial dry dog food, which had a protein level generally considered to be insufficient for ferrets (Nguyen *et al.*, 1979).

Clinical signs

There will be frequent urination, licking at the perineal area, dysuria, and sometimes haemorrhage. Straining to pass urine can lead to a rectal or vaginal prolapse. Sometimes there is complete obstruction or may be paradoxical incontinence, and urine dribbling can cause the ventral abdomen to become wet. If untreated, a urethral blockage can lead to uraemia and death.

Diagnosis

The clinical signs will be suggestive, and the diagnosis can be confirmed by radiography. Sometimes the stones or enlarged bladder may be palpable on clinical examination.

Treatment and control

If there is complete urethral obstruction, this must be relieved as soon as possible. Catheterisation of the male ferret is difficult, since the j-shaped os penis prevents the easy passage of a catheter. Try anaesthetising the animal with isoflurane to get maximum muscle relaxation before inserting the catheter. If the catheter cannot pass, insert it as far as possible into the urethra and flush with sterile saline to try to force the stone back into the bladder from where it can be removed. If this is unsuccessful, a perineal urethrostomy will be required. Cystocentesis can provide temporary relief until the blockage is cleared. Insert a needle through the abdominal wall into the bladder under aseptic conditions as in cats, taking care to leave some urine in the bladder to prevent the needle causing damage to the bladder wall. If there is no obstruction, stabilise the animal and perform a cystotomy to remove the stones. Flush the bladder carefully afterwards, and give i.v. fluids for at least 24 hours post operatively. Give the animal potentiated sulphonamides to kill urease producing bacteria such as *Staphylococcus* or *Proteus* which can raise the pH.

Uroliths can be largely prevented by improving the diet. Gradually replace the diet with a better, animal protein based one over a period of seven to ten days, provide plenty of water and reduce the dietary ash level. Diets which dissolve stones may be of benefit, e.g. feline s/d (Hills Pet Nutrition), although the protein level may not be sufficient for long term use in ferrets.

Cystitis and pyelonephritis

Bacterial urinary tract infections are common, particularly in female ferrets, and are often associated with uroliths. Organisms such as *E. coli* or *Staphylococcus aureus* are often isolated. These infections may be subclinical, but can lead to ascending urinary tract infections or septicaemia, resulting in pyelonephritis. The clinical signs are fever, anorexia, depression, and severe cases may end in renal failure. Diagnosis may be made by urinalysis, which will show blood, white blood cells and tubular casts as well as bacteria. Pyelonephritis can be hard to distinguish from lower urinary tract infections. Treat with supportive therapy, fluids and antibiotics (after culture and sensitivity) for seven to ten days.

Cystic kidneys

Cysts are often seen in the kidneys as incidental findings during abdominal ultrasound or post mortem examination. Cysts may be single or multiple, and affect one of both kidneys. Usually no clinical signs are associated with these. True polycystic disease is rare: several cysts may be found throughout the kidney parenchyma and other organs such as the liver, and the enlarged, irregular kidneys may be palpable on clinical examination. Animals with polycystic disease may present with renal failure, and serum biochemistry should be done to evaluate renal function. No treatment is required, unless the cyst is large or painful, in which case unilateral nephrectomy can be performed provided the remaining kidney is functioning.

Hydronephrosis

This is very rare. The animal presents with progressive abdominal distension in the absence of other signs. This can occur if the ureter is inadvertently ligated during ovariohysterectomy. Diagnosis may be made on the clinical signs and radiography, serum biochemistry and urinalysis. A fine needle aspirate from the mass will confirm the presence of urine. Remove the affected kidney.

Chronic interstitial nephritis

This is a fairly common finding in older ferrets. The aetiology is unsure, but the high protein diet which ferrets need may be a factor. In advanced cases there will be polyuria, polydipsia and weight loss related to renal insufficiency. Some practitioners recommend reducing the protein level in the diet for ferrets over three years of age to reduce the incidence of this.

Glomerulonephropathy

This can occur due to immune complex deposition in cases of Aleutian disease.

Prostatic squamous metaplasia and prostatic cysts

Adrenal-related endocrinopathy often results in the production of oestrogens, which in the male cause squamous metaplasia in the region of the prostate. Secretory material and keratin accumulations result in the formation of multiple, fluctuant cysts around the bladder neck, which can cause dysuria and urethral blockage and may become infected. The diagnosis of adrenocortical disease is discussed in Chapter 9. Prostatic cysts can be palpable on clinical examination, and contrast radiography may show an irregular blockage around the neck of the bladder. Removing the affected adrenal gland(s) will usually result in resolution of the prostatic cysts, or they can be drained or removed surgically.

Neoplasia

Reproductive tract neoplasms are common in entire ferrets, but are obviously rare in neutered animals, although ovarian remnant tumours can still occur. Ovarian tumours may contain mixed cell types, may be bilateral, and include granulosa cell tumours, fibrosarcomas, dysgerminoma, leiomyomas, teratomas, thecomas and carcinomas (see Plate 15). Affected animals may be asymptomatic or present with ill thrift, persistent oestrus, alopecia, anaemia or palpable abdominal masses. Ovariohysterectomy is usually curative.

Males may develop interstitial cell or Sertoli cell tumours, and these usually cause no signs other than swelling of one or both testicles. Removal of the affected testicle will be curative. Feminisation with Sertoli cell tumours is rare. Cryptorchid testicles are prone to becoming neoplastic and should be removed.

Urinary tract neoplasms are comparatively rare, but occur occasionally in mature animals. Transitional cell carcinomas produce signs similar to chronic cystitis, and may be diagnosed by radiography and by identifying neoplastic cells on urinalysis. Renal carcinomas may be palpable on clinical examination, and often there are no associated clinical signs. Both of these tumours are malignant with a poor prognosis: transitional cell carcinomas infiltrate widely into the bladder wall, and pulmonary metastases are common with renal carcinomas.

Reference

Nguyen, H.T., Moreland, A.F. and Shields, R.P. (1979) Urolithiasis in ferrets (*Mustela putorius*). *Laboratory Animal Science*, **29**, pp. 243–5.

14 NUTRITIONAL DISEASES

The nutritional needs of the ferret have not been extensively studied, however much information has been obtained by extrapolating from the dietary needs of mink and from observing the effects of different diets on colonies of ferrets. Nutrition is discussed in more detail in Chapter 3. Briefly, ferrets have a short intestine and rapid gut transit time, and food passes right through the intestines in about three hours, so there is little time for bacterial or enzymatic digestion or the synthesis and absorption of complex molecules. They need diets which are high in protein, and low in fibre, and frequent small meals appear to be best. Ferrets eat to calorie requirements, so on diets with a low protein level they will become protein deficient, leading to poor reproductive performance, and if the energy density is low they can develop metabolic disorders such as pregnancy toxaemia (see Chapter 11).

Several specific nutritional diseases have been identified in ferrets, but there are no doubt many more which have yet to be discovered.

Nutritional steatitis (yellow fat disease)

Aetiology and pathogenesis

This disease occurs if animals are fed diets which are high in polyunsaturated fatty acids (PUFAs), such as those containing high proportions of oily marine fish such as tuna, or if they contain freezer-burned horsemeat. PUFAs lead to oxidation of the fat both within the food source and in the animal, causing oxidative injury to the tissues. If the diet is low in vitamin E, this can precipitate the disease at a lower level of PUFAs. Dietary vitamin E protects against oxidative injury.

Clinical signs

Signs are seen mainly in young, rapidly growing animals. They may be found dead, or depressed, lethargic, anorexic and reluctant to move. On examination, there are firm, diffuse painful swellings in the inguinal and flank regions. Sometimes there will be dyspnoea, hind leg weakness, diarrhoea or black, tarry faeces. On post mortem examination, the fat is yellow brown in colour with a coarse granular texture.

Diagnosis

The diagnosis can be made on the history and clinical signs.

Treatment and control

Give any affected animals 10 mg vitamin E daily by subcutaneous injection for two days and change the diet to one lower in PUFAs. Then, add 30 mg vitamin E per ferret per day to the diet, reducing to 15 mg after five days and then to 10 mg after another five days, keeping it at this level for maintenance.

   To prevent the disease, careful management of the diet for growing animals is needed. Diets which contain higher levels of PUFAs will need correspondingly higher vitamin E levels, sometimes as much as 150 mg vitamin E per ferret per day. If possible, avoid giving growing ferrets diets which may contain rancid fats or high levels of PUFAs.

Osteodystrophy
(see Chapter 8)

Aetiology and pathogenesis

This has been observed in ferrets fed on an all meat diet with no calcium supplementation, and is essentially caused by hyperphos-phorosis. The calcium–phosphorus imbalance leads to nutritional secondary hyperparathyroidism, and poor calcification of the bones. True rickets, due to vitamin D deficiency, is rare.

Clinical signs

The disease is seen mainly in growing animals in the 6–12 week age group. Often, the first sign the owner notices is the sudden death of several apparently well-nourished kits in one litter. When alive, these animals have soft, deformed bones and typically they are unable to stand, moving with a seal-like gait on their bellies with front legs abducted. Affected animals need urgent dietary correction, and may still be left with deformed limbs and vertebrae (see Plate 10). The ferret can survive if this occurs, but may not be sufficiently mobile to continue working.

Diagnosis

Diagnosis can be made on the history and clinical signs, and confirmed by radiography.

Treatment

Correct the diet of such animals at once, by the addition of balanced mineral and vitamin supplements such as SA-37 (Intervet) or Pet-Cal tablets (Pfizer) to the diet, alternatively 5–10% ground bone, 2% bone flour, or 2% dicalcium phosphate can be used. The condition can be prevented by making sure the calcium:phosphorus ratio in the diet is 1:1.

Thiamine deficiency
(see Chapter 8)

This occurs if animals are fed diets high in thiaminase, such as eggs, frozen day-old chicks or raw fish (e.g. herring, mullet, sprats, dogfish, squid, carp, crabs and mussels). Signs are most often seen in the 8–12 week age group, and include lethargy, anorexia, hind limb weakness and convulsions. Death may follow within two to three days. Give injections of vitamin B-complex, 5 mg daily for three days. Signs may resolve within hours of treatment.

Zinc toxicity
(see Chapter 8)

Ferrets are very susceptible to zinc toxicity, levels above 500 ppm causing clinical signs in animals of any age. Animals which are fed from galvanised dishes may develop the condition if the process used to clean the dishes results in the deposition of zinc oxide on the dish. Gastric haemorrhages and depression of the bone marrow lead to anaemia, and nephrosis and liver failure lead to uraemia, coma and death. Clinically affected animals have pale mucous membranes and are in poor condition, and there may be lethargy, anorexia, anaemia and hind limb weakness. On post mortem, the liver is orange in colour and the kidneys are pale and soft. There is no treatment, and the prognosis is poor. Ferrets should not be given galvanised water and food bowls.

Biotin deficiency
(see Chapter 10)

Biotin deficiency is seen in diets high in raw eggs, which contain avidin. This binds to biotin preventing its absorption and leading to clinical signs. Affected animals may develop alopecia. Treat affected animals by removing or boiling the eggs, or by adding biotin supplements to the diet.

Salt poisoning

This has been seen in ferrets fed a diet of fish stored in brine. Affected animals become depressed and develop spasms within 24–96 hours after ingestion of the salty diet; death follows shortly after. Treat affected animals by removing the salty food from the diet and providing ample fresh water.

15 NEOPLASIA

Reports of spontaneous neoplasia in ferrets are relatively rare, although the incidence has been increasing since the first reported case in 1944. This paucity of reports is probably because laboratory ferrets are short lived and do not have time to develop neoplasia, because pet ferrets have been few and far between until recently, or because owners are reluctant to submit pet or working ferrets for full post mortem examination and histology. It was believed that ferrets had a genetic resistance to the development of neoplasia, but this is probably not the case. In the USA, the incidence appears to be much greater than in Europe, adrenocortical neoplasia, lymphoma or insulinoma occurring in a high proportion of older ferrets. There are many possible explanations for this difference, including:

(1) Genetic predisposition. In the USA, there are many closed colonies which may result in genetic factors being concentrated. Production in Europe and Australia is much less intensive.

(2) Early neutering, at five to six weeks of age. This is commonly practised in the USA and may interfere with the development of the endocrine system in these very immature animals.

(3) Lack of natural light. Ferrets are very sensitive to photoperiod, and the effects of long-term artificial lighting are unknown. It is common for ferrets in Europe and Australia to be kept outdoors under natural light, with seasonal variation.

(4) Diet. Commercial processed diets may contain too little protein, excess carbohydrate or other components which could be involved in the development of neoplasia.

(5) Infection. Retroviral causes have been postulated for lymphoma.

Reports vary as to which neoplasm is the most common. In the USA, the commonest neoplasms (in order of decreasing significance) are probably insulinoma, lymphoma, adrenocortical neoplasia, and skin neoplasms, but in Europe the most common are tumours of the reproductive tract, lymphoid system and skin. It is quite common for two or more different neoplasms to be found in the same animal. Primary neoplasms have been reported in all organ systems except the cardiovascular system, although tumours of the respiratory tract and central nervous system are extremely rare. Nearly half of all tumours reported have been classified as malignant, which (although locally invasive) rarely metastasise in the ferret.

Most cases occur in ferrets between four and seven years of age, but some have occurred in animals less than one year old. The clinician should be aware that ferrets with neoplasms are increasingly likely to present themselves in the consulting room, and owners are increasingly likely to want the best treatment for their ferret. Always advise them that any neoplasm has the potential to metastasise, so be sure to check the whole animal for secondary tumours, and give a guarded prognosis until a mass has been confirmed as benign. It is rare for abdominal tumours to spread into the chest cavity, and vice versa. Resection of the tumour if possible is usually the best treatment, however recurrences at the site or in local lymph nodes may occur. Neoplasms in the distal limb may best be treated by amputation, and ferrets can do well with only three legs.

Neoplasms occurring in specific organ systems are covered in the relevant chapters: this chapter will concentrate on those tumours which do not fall into any particular category.

Lymphosarcoma

Aetiology and pathogenesis

Lymphosarcoma is the commonest haematopoietic neoplasm in ferrets, and it follows the same patterns of distribution as in dogs and cats. There may be solid tumours in organs such as the liver, spleen and lymph nodes, disseminated lesions throughout the lymph nodes, spleen, thymus, liver, meninges, thorax, or abdomen, or leukaemic forms affecting the circulating blood. Affected animals tend to fall into two groups, animals less than one year old which tend to develop an acute lymphoblastic form with thymic involvement, and animals over two years old which develop a more chronic lymphocytic disease and often show lymphadenopathy. Males and females are equally affected, as are neutered and entire animals. The leukaemic form is relatively rare, but may be seen in the later stages of both juvenile and adult forms of the disease.

The aetiology of lymphosarcoma has not been fully elucidated, but there have been suggestions of an infectious cause, since it is common to find clusters of cases, and lymphosarcoma has been transmitted experimentally from one ferret to others by both cells and cell-free inocula. Infection with Aleutian disease virus causes hypergammaglobulinaemia and this has been postulated to interfere with the immune system leading to lymphosarcoma, although this has not been proven. Other reports describe the isolation of reverse transcriptase from splenocytes and mononuclear cells in affected ferrets suggesting a retroviral aetiology, although no agent has yet been identified. *Helicobacter mustelae* has been implicated in cases of gastric lymphosarcoma.

Clinical signs

The clinical signs depend upon the site of the lesion and are often non-specific. In juvenile animals which develop the acute lymphoblastic form, large immature lymphocytes rapidly infiltrate the viscera, causing signs depending upon the organs affected. Animals exhibit a rapidly progressive loss of condition, with anorexia, weakness and lethargy. Sometimes animals develop a sudden pyrexia and collapse. Dyspnoea is common, due to an enlarging thymic mass and pleural effusion, but lymphadenopathy is rare (see Plate 16). Radiography may show a mediastinal mass and pleural effusion. Young animals are more likely to die from the disease than adults.

Some cases in animals aged less than one year present with signs similar to those of a gastric foreign body, with palpable masses in the abdomen due to involvement of the mesenteric lymph nodes.

In adults, small, mature lymphocytes infiltrate the peripheral and mesenteric nodes, gradually destroying the nodal architecture. Usually there is peripheral and visceral lymphadenopathy, with some organ involvement later in the course of disease. The disease is insidious and chronic in onset, and there may be no signs until the disease is advanced. Animals may have cycles of anorexia, weight loss and lethargy over months or years. There may be recurrent upper respiratory or gastrointestinal infections, diarrhoea or vomiting, dyspnoea, jaundice, or posterior paralysis. They may respond to antibiotics initially, only to relapse when treatment finishes. Corticosteroid therapy may produce a longer period of remission: consider lymphosarcoma as a differential in animals which respond to corticosteroids. Splenomegaly is common in animals with lymphosarcoma, but often this is due to extramedullary haemopoiesis rather than infiltration with malignant lymphocytes.

Diagnosis

Diagnosis can be difficult, since the signs are very vague and lymphadenopathy can occur for many reasons. Lymphosarcoma may be diagnosed provisionally on the history and clinical signs, and confirmed by cytology or histology on blood, tissue aspirates or biopsies of solid tumours. There may be changes in the serum biochemistry depending on the organs affected. Haematology may be normal, or there may be mild anaemia with an increased or decreased white cell count. Lymphocytosis is common, although older animals with chronic disease are often lymphopenic. Do not make the diagnosis on the basis of peripheral lymphocytosis alone, since this can occur for many reasons and is often unrelated to lymphoproliferative disease. The lymphocyte count can be used as a screening procedure however. If the absolute lymphocyte count is more than 3500/mm^3 or the relative count more than 60%, this is suggestive of lymphosarcoma and other tests are then required to confirm the diagnosis. Repeat the haematology after three or four weeks, and if there is still a lymphocytosis, perform a lymph node biopsy (see below) or bone marrow biopsy (see Chapter 17). The latter is particularly useful if there is anaemia or leucopenia, or if there are abnormal cells in peripheral blood.

When taking a needle biopsy from a peripheral lymph node, it can be hard to locate the node accurately since they lie within fat pads. An excisional biopsy is more accurate. The popliteal lymph node is easy to biopsy, and is located on the caudal thigh in a fat pad midway between hip and stifle. The tan-coloured, round or oblong node can be separated from the fat using blunt dissection. Lymph node biopsies can be taken during exploratory laparotomy; however the gastric lymph node is often enlarged for other reasons and may not be a good site for sampling.

Treatment and control

The choices for treatment are surgery, chemotherapy, radiotherapy or combinations of these. However, the prognosis is guarded, and this should be discussed with the owner in detail before any treatment is attempted. Even if there appears to be only one organ affected, the disease is likely to be systemic, although the prognosis is improved if the affected organ can be removed. Some forms of lymphosarcoma can be treated using chemotherapeutic regimes similar to those used in dogs or cats, with up to 70% of animals going into remission. The chance of a successful outcome is greater if the animal is presented early in the course of the disease, if aggressive therapy is given, and if the initial response to treatment is good.

Animals with lymphosarcoma affecting the mediastinum, spleen, skin and peripheral lymph nodes often respond favourably to therapy, but a poor response is usually seen in animals with disease affecting the liver, intestine, solitary lymph nodes, multiple abdominal organs or the bone marrow. The prognosis is also poor in animals with intercurrent disease, or in those which have been pretreated with prednisolone. So before considering treatment, evaluate the animal to assess its general condition and the stage of the disease. Take blood samples for full haematology, and serum biochemistry to asses major organ function. Take x-rays to look for dissemination or lung metastases, and a bone marrow biopsy to assess the animal's ability to withstand chemotherapy: if more than 50% of bone marrow cells show signs of malignancy then the animal will probably not withstand treatment. Continue to monitor the animal's blood profile and general condition throughout treatment, and stop if the white cell count falls below $1500/mm^3$, or the PCV falls below 30%. Treatment can be restarted once the blood picture returns to normal.

The best treatment regimes involve using vincristine, asparaginase, cyclophosphamide, doxorubicin and prednisolone in combinations, over a 14 week period (see Table 15.1). Always follow health and safety guidelines when working with these agents. The implantation of a vascular access port can facilitate the repeated administration of intravenous drugs. This consists of a plastic dome-shaped reservoir chamber with a self sealing silicone diaphragm on top. Connected to this is a silicone cannula, which can be implanted into the jugular vein. The chamber is implanted under the skin over

Table 15.1 Suggested protocol for use of cytotoxic agents in lymphosarcoma.

Drug	Dose
Prednisolone	2 mg/kg daily for three months
Vincristine	0.75 mg/m² i.v. once weekly for up to 4 weeks*
Cyclophosphamide	50 mg/m² p.o. weekly for four weeks

* For 400–500 g female, give 0.05 mg, for 1 kg female, give 0.07 mg, for 1.5 kg male, give 0.1 mg. Anaesthetise the animal with isoflurane and give the vincristine slowly via a cephalic intravenous cannula or vascular access port. Accidental perivascular administration of vincristine results in severe tissue necrosis.

the back, and drugs can be given i.v. by giving them percutaneously into the chamber. These are available from Sandown Scientific, 11 Copsem Drive, Esher, Surrey, KT10 9HD.

The protocol can be modified to include other treatments in addition to or instead of the above. Doxorubicin at 1 mg/kg i.v. every 21 days for five treatments alone or with orthovoltage radiation can be successful. Alternatively, vincristine, cyclophosphamide and doxorubicin can be used in sequence weekly for the 14 week period of treatment in conjunction with prednisolone. Asparaginase at 400 i.u./kg i.p. given once in the first week may be beneficial. Cytotoxic agents have numerous side effects, including lethargy, posterior paresis, anorexia, vomiting, hair loss (often just the whiskers), dyspnoea and collapse. These may manifest from two days to two weeks after treatment starts.

Prednisolone alone can produce an initial improvement in clinical signs, but the disease is likely to recur within four to six weeks, and it will then be refractory to treatment with other agents. However, this may still be worth considering as a palliative treatment in animals which are poor candidates for cytotoxic agents. Another treatment which may be beneficial for these animals is vitamin C, which has some antineoplastic properties in man. Try 50–100 mg/kg p.o. twice daily.

In all cases, it is important that the animal is given excellent nutrition. Give the animal a good quality diet high in meat protein and fat, supplemented with e.g. Nutri-plus gel (Virbac).

Even with a good response to therapy, the disease is likely to recur, and animals should be reassessed every three months or so. Periods of remission can last for a few months to several years.

Other haematopoietic neoplasms

Other variants of haematopoietic neoplasms reported include myeloid leukaemia, erythroleukaemia and megakaryocytic leukaemia. Mycosis fungoides is a variant of lymphosarcoma which presents as a dermatitis. Histiocytic tumours and splenic haemangiosarcomas have also been identified.

Myeloma

Myelomas arise from plasma cells in the bone marrow, and may present with many signs depending on the site of the lesion. They may affect one or more bones, including the vertebrae, pelvis, skull and limbs. Animals may present with pain, lameness, fractures, paralysis or even haemorrhagic diathesis. Radiography shows focal osteolysis without bony sclerosis.

Thymoma

These are uncommon leaf shaped tan or red brown masses found in the cranial mediastinum visible on radiography. They may cause dyspnoea and ventricular enlargement, vomiting, lethargy and coughing. Oesophageal enlargement can occur anterior to the mass.

Other miscellaneous neoplasms

A rapidly growing, red, firm, hairless mass protruding from the ear canal in an animal with vestibular signs was identified as a complex ceruminous gland adenocarcinoma.

Myelolipomas consist of variable proportions of adipose and haemopoietic elements, and are an incidental finding at post mortem in humans and many species of animal, including the ferret. They may be found as white or yellow nodules with a waxy or fatty appearance.

Further reading

Chapter 6

Bernard, S.L., Gorham, J.R. and Ryland, R.M. (1984) Biology and diseases of ferrets. In: J.G. Fox, B.J. Cohen and F.M. Loew (eds). *Laboratory Animal Medicine*. Academic Press, Orlando, pp. 386–97.

Burke, T.J. (1988) Common diseases and medical management of ferrets. In: E.R. Jacobson and G.V. Kollias (eds). *Exotic Animals*. Churchill Livingstone, Edinburgh, pp. 247–60.

Fox, J.G. (1998) Bacterial and mycoplasmal diseases. In: J.G. Fox (ed.). *Biology and Diseases of the Ferret*. 2nd edn. Williams and Wilkins, Baltimore, pp. 321–54.

Fox, J.G. (1998) Mycotic diseases. In: J.G. Fox (ed.). *Biology and Diseases of the Ferret*. 2nd edn. Williams and Wilkins, Baltimore, pp. 393–403.

Fox, J.G., Pearson, R.C. and Gorham, J.R. (1998) Viral diseases. In: J.G. Fox (ed.). *Biology and Diseases of the Ferret*. 2nd edn. Williams and Wilkins, Baltimore, pp. 355–74.

Oxenham, M. (1991) Ferrets. In: P.H. Beynon and J.E. Cooper (eds). *Manual of Exotic Pets*. British Small Animal Veterinary Association, Cheltenham, pp. 97–109.

Rosenthal, K.L. (1997) Respiratory diseases. In: E.V. Hillyer and K.E. Quesenberry (eds). *Ferrets, Rabbits, and Rodents: Clinical Medicine and Surgery*. W.B. Saunders, Philadelphia, pp. 77–84.

Russell, P.H. and Edington, N. (1985) *Veterinary Viruses*. Burlington Press, Cambridge.

Ryland, L.M. and Gorham, J.R. (1978) The ferret and its diseases. *Journal of the American Veterinary Medical Association*, **173**(9), pp. 1154–8.

Taylor, M. (1992) Diseases of ferrets. *Veterinary Technician*, **13**, pp. 56–60.

Williams, B.H. (1996) Pathology of the domestic ferret. Proceedings of a C.L. Davis Foundation European Symposium.

Chapter 7

Bell, J.A. (1997) *Helicobacter mustelae* gastritis, proliferative bowel disease and eosinophilic gastroenteritis. In: E.V. Hillyer and K.E.

Quesenberry (eds). *Ferrets, Rabbits, and Rodents: Clinical Medicine and Surgery.* W.B. Saunders, Philadelphia, pp. 37–43.

Bishop, Y. (ed.) (1996) *The Veterinary Formulary.* Royal Pharmaceutical Society of Great Britain and British Veterinary Association, London.

Brown, S.A. (1998) Gastrointestinal diseases of ferrets. Paper given at BSAVA Congress, Birmingham, UK.

Fox, J.G. (1998) Bacterial and mycoplasmal diseases. In: J.G. Fox (ed.). *Biology and Diseases of the Ferret.* 2nd edn. Williams and Wilkins, Baltimore, pp. 321–54.

Fox, J.G. (1998) Diseases of the gastrointestinal system. In: J.G. Fox (ed.). *Biology and Diseases of the Ferret.* 2nd edn. Williams and Wilkins, Baltimore, pp. 273–90.

Fox, J.G. (1998) Parasitic diseases. In: J.G. Fox (ed.). *Biology and Diseases of the Ferret.* 2nd edn. Williams and Wilkins, Baltimore, pp. 375–91.

Harms, C.A. and Andrews, G.A. (1993) Megaoesophagus in a domestic ferret. *Laboratory Animal Science*, **43**(5), pp. 506–8.

Hoefer, H.L. (1997) Gastrointestinal diseases. In: E.V. Hillyer and K.E. Quesenberry (eds). *Ferrets, Rabbits, and Rodents: Clinical Medicine and Surgery.* W.B. Saunders, Philadelphia, pp. 26–36.

Li, X., Pang, J. and Fox, J.G. (1996) Coinfection with intracellular *Desulfovibrio* species and coccidia in ferrets with proliferative bowel disease. *Laboratory Animal Science*, **46**(5), pp. 569–71.

Marini, R.P., Fox, J.G., Taylor, N.S., Yan, L., McColm, A. and Williamson, R. (1997) Evaluation of ranitidine-bismuth-citrate and clarithromycin combination treatment for eradication of *Helicobacter mustelae* from ferrets. *Laboratory Animal Science*, **47**, p. 434.

Moody, K.D., Bowman, T.A. and Lang, C.M. (1985) Laboratory management of the ferret for biomedical research. *Laboratory Animal Science*, **35**(3), pp. 272–9.

Rosenthal, K. (1994) Ferrets. *Veterinary Clinics of North America: Small Animal Practice*, **24**, pp. 1–23.

Williams, B.H. (1996) Pathology of the domestic ferret. Proceedings of a C.L. Davis Foundation European Symposium.

Chapter 8

Antinoff, N. (1997) Musculoskeletal and neurologic disorders. In: E.V. Hillyer and K.E. Quesenberry (eds). *Ferrets, Rabbits, and Rodents:*

Clinical Medicine and Surgery. W.B. Saunders, Philadelphia, pp. 126–30.

Bernard, S.L., Gorham, J.R. and Ryland, R.M. (1984) Biology and diseases of ferrets: IV–VI diseases. In: J.G. Fox, B.J. Cohen and F.M. Loew (eds). *Laboratory Animal Medicine*. Academic Press, Orlando, pp. 389–97.

Besch-Williford, C.L. (1987) Biology and medicine of the ferret. *Veterinary Clinics of North America: Small Animal Practice*, **17**, pp. 1155–83.

Burke, T.J. (1988) Common diseases and medical management of ferrets. In: E.R. Jacobson and G.V. Kollias (eds). *Exotic Animals*. Churchill Livingstone, Edinburgh, pp. 247–60.

Fox, J.G. (1998) Bacterial and mycoplasmal diseases. In: J.G. Fox (ed.). *Biology and Diseases of the Ferret*. 2nd edn. Williams and Wilkins, Baltimore, pp. 321–54.

Fox, J.G. (1998) Other systemic diseases. In: J.G. Fox (ed.) *Biology and Diseases of the Ferret*. 2nd edn. Williams and Wilkins, Baltimore, pp. 307–20.

Fox, J.G., Pearson, R.C. and Gorham, J.R. (1998) Viral diseases. In: J.G. Fox (ed.). *Biology and Diseases of the Ferret*. 2nd edn. Williams and Wilkins, Baltimore, pp. 355–74.

Gill, J. (1989) Outbreak of possible thiamine deficiency in farmed ferrets. *Surveillance – Wellington*, **16**, pp. 16–17.

Harrison, S.G. and Borland, E.D. (1973) Deaths in ferrets (*Mustela putorius*) due to *Clostridium botulinum* type C. *Veterinary Record*, **93**, pp. 576–7.

Lloyd, M.H. and Wood, C.M. (1996) Synovial sarcoma in a ferret. *Veterinary Record*, **139**, pp. 627–8.

Okada, H.M., Chihaya, Y. and Matsukawa, K. (1987) Thiamine deficiency encephalopathy in foxes and mink. *Veterinary Pathology*, **24**, pp. 180–2.

Oxenham, M. (1990) Aleutian disease in the ferret. *Veterinary Record*, **126**, p. 585.

Oxenham, M. (1991) Ferrets. In: P.H. Beynon and J.E. Cooper (eds). *Manual of Exotic Pets*. British Small Animal Veterinary Association, Cheltenham, pp. 97–110.

Porter, H.G., Porter, D.D. and Larsen, A.E. (1982) Aleutian disease in ferrets. *Infection and Immunity*, **36**, pp. 379–86.

Porter, V. and Brown, N. (1997) *The Complete Book of Ferrets*. D & M Publications, Bedford.

Rosenthal, K. (1994) Ferrets. *Veterinary Clinics of North America: Small Animal Practice*, **24**, pp. 1–23.

Stewart, J.D. and Rozengurt, N. (1993) Aleutian disease in the ferret. *Veterinary Record*, **133**, p. 172.

Williams, B.H. (1996) Pathology of a domestic ferret. Proceedings of a C.L. Davis Foundation European Symposium.

Wolfensohn, S.E. and Lloyd, M.H. (1994) Aleutian disease in laboratory ferrets. *Veterinary Record*, **134**, p. 100.

Chapter 9

Bernard, S.L., Gorham, J.R. and Ryland, R.M. (1984) Biology and diseases of ferrets: IV–VI Diseases. In: J.G. Fox, B.J. Cohen and F.M. Loew (eds). *Laboratory Animal Medicine*. Academic Press, Orlando, pp. 389–97.

Brown, S.A. (1998) Diagnosis and management of neoplastic diseases in ferrets. Paper given at BSAVA Congress, Birmingham, UK.

Caplan, E.R., Peterson, M.E., Mullen, H.S. *et al.* (1996) Diagnosis and treatment of insulin-secreting pancreatic islet cell tumours in ferrets: 57 cases (1986–1994). *Journal of the American Veterinary Medical Association*, **209**, pp. 1741–5.

Ehrhart, N., Withrow, S.J., Ehrhart, E.J. *et al.* (1996) Pancreatic beta cell tumours in ferrets: 20 cases (1986–1994). *Journal of the American Veterinary Medical Association*, **209**, pp. 1737–40.

Fox, J.G. and Marini, R.P. (1998) Diseases of the endocrine system. In: J.G. Fox (ed.). *Biology and Diseases of the Ferret*. 2nd edn. Williams and Wilkins, Baltimore, pp. 291–305.

Fox, J.G., Pearson, R.G. and Bell, J.A. (1998) Diseases of the genito-urinary system. In: J.G. Fox (ed.). *Biology and Diseases of the Ferret*. 2nd edn. Williams and Wilkins, Baltimore, pp. 231–46.

Garibaldi, B.A., Pecquet-Goad, M.E. and Fox, J.G. (1987) Serum cortisol radioimmunoassay values in the normal ferret and response to ACTH stimulation and dexamethasone suppression tests. *Laboratory Animal Science*, **37**, p. 545.

Hillyer, E.V. (1997) Urogenital diseases. In: E.V. Hillyer and K.E. Quesenberry (eds), *Ferrets, Rabbits, and Rodents: Clinical Medicine and Surgery*. W.B. Saunders, Philadelphia, pp. 44–52.

Kociba, G.J. and Caputo, C.A. (1981) Aplastic anaemia associated with oestrus in pet ferrets. *Journal of the American Veterinary Medical Association*, **178**, pp. 1293–4.

Nelson, R.W., Turnwald, G.H. and Willard, M.D. (1994) Endocrine, metabolic and lipid disorders. In: M.D. Willard, H. Tvedten and G.H. Turnwald (eds), *Small Animal Clinical Diagnosis by Laboratory Methods*, 2nd edn. W.B. Saunders Co, Philadelphia, pp. 147–78.

Oxenham, M. (1990) Oestrus control in the ferret. *Veterinary Record*, **126**, pp. 148.

Oxenham, M. (1991) Ferrets. In: P.H. Beynon and J.E. Cooper (eds), *Manual of Exotic Pets*. British Small Animal Veterinary Association, Cheltenham, pp. 97–109.

Quesenberry, K.E. (1997) Endocrine diseases: Part I. In: E.V. Hillyer and K.E. Quesenberry (eds), *Ferrets, Rabbits, and Rodents: Clinical Medicine and Surgery*. W.B. Saunders, Philadelphia, pp. 85–90.

Rosenthal, K. (1994) Ferrets. *Veterinary Clinics of North America: Small Animal Practice*, **24**, pp. 1–23.

Taylor, M. (1992) Diseases for ferrets. *Veterinary Technician*, **13**, pp. 56–60.

Williams, B.H. (1996) Pathology of the Domestic Ferret. Proceedings of a C.L. Davis Foundation European Symposium.

Chapter 10

Bernard, S.L., Gorham, J.R. and Ryland, R.M. (1984) Biology and diseases of ferrets: IV–VI diseases. In: J.G. Fox, B.J. Cohen and F.M. Loew (eds). *Laboratory Animal Medicine*. Academic Press, Orlando, pp. 389–97.

Besch-Williford, C.L. (1987) Biology and medicine of the ferret. *Veterinary Clinics of North America: Small Animal Practice*, **17**, pp. 1155–83.

Burke, T.J. (1988) Common diseases and medical management of ferrets. In: E.R. Jacobson and G.V. Kollias (eds). *Exotic Animals*. Churchill Livingstone, Edinburgh, pp. 247–60.

Cooper, J.E. (1990) Skin diseases of ferrets. *The Veterinary Annual*, **30**, pp. 325–34.

Fox, J.G. (1998) Bacterial and mycoplasmal diseases. In: J.G. Fox (ed.). *Biology and Diseases of the Ferrets*. 2nd edn. Williams and Wilkins, Baltimore, pp. 321–54.

Fox, J.G. (1998) Mycotic diseases. In: J.G. Fox (ed.). *Biology and Diseases of the Ferret*. 2nd edn. Williams and Wilkins, Baltimore, pp. 393–403.

Fox, J.G. (1998) Parasitic diseases. In: J.G. Fox (ed.). *Biology and Diseases of the Ferret*. 2nd edn. Williams and Wilkins, Baltimore, pp. 375–91.

Gyles, C.L. (1993) *Nocardia, actinomyces, dermatophilus*. In: C.L. Gyles and C.O. Thoen (eds). *Pathogenesis of Bacterial Infections in Animals*. Iowa State University Press, Iowa City, pp. 124–32.

Orcutt, C. (1997) Dermatologic diseases. In: E.V. Hillyer and K.E. Quesenberry (eds). *Ferrets, Rabbits, and Rodents: Clinical Medicine and Surgery*. W.B. Saunders, Philadelphia, pp. 115–25.

Oxenham, M. (1991) Ferrets. In: P.H. Beynon and J.E. Cooper (eds). *Manual of Exotic Pets*. British Small Animal Veterinary Association, Cheltenham, pp. 97–109.

Porter, V. and Brown, N. (1997) *The Complete Book of Ferrets*. D & M Publications, Bedford.

Rosenthal, K. (1994) Ferrets. *Veterinary Clinics of North America: Small Animal Practice*, **24**, pp. 1–23.

Soulsby, E.J.L. (1982) *Helminths, Arthropods and Protozoa of Domesticated Animals*. 7th edn., Baillière Tindall, London.

Williams, B.H. (1996) Pathology of the domestic ferret. Proceedings of a C.L. Davis Foundation European Symposium.

Chapter 11

Bell, J.A. (1997) Periparturient and neonatal diseases. In: E.V. Hillyer and K.E. Quesenberry (eds). *Ferrets, Rabbits, and Rodents: Clinical Medicine and Surgery*. W.B. Saunders, Philadelphia, pp. 53–62.

Fox, J.G. and Bell, J.A. (1998) Growth, reproduction and breeding. In: J.G. Fox (ed.). *Biology and Diseases of the Ferret*. 2nd edn. Williams and Wilkins, Baltimore, pp. 211–30.

Fox, J.G., Pearson, R.G. and Bell, J.A. (1998) Diseases of the genitourinary system. In: J.G. Fox (ed.). *Biology and Diseases of the Ferret*. 2nd edn. Williams and Wilkins, Baltimore, pp. 231–46.

Huerkamp, M.J., Murray, K.A. and Orosz, S.E. (1996) Guinea pigs. In: K. Laber-Laird, M.M. Swindle and P.A. Flecknell (eds). *Handbook of Rodent and Rabbit Medicine*. Pergamon Press, Oxford, pp. 91–151.

Oxenham, M. (1991) Ferrets. In: P.H. Beynon and J.E. Cooper (eds). *Manual of Exotic Pets*. British Small Animal Veterinary Association, Cheltenham, pp. 97–109.

Porter, V. and Brown, N. (1997) *The Complete Book of Ferrets*. D & M Publications, Bedford.

Randolph, R.W. (1989) Medical and surgical care in the pet ferret. In: R.W. Kirk (ed.). *Current Veterinary Therapy X*. W.B. Saunders, Philadelphia, pp. 765–75.

Smith, D.A. and Burgmann, P.M. (1997) Formulary. In: E.V. Hillyer and K.E. Quesenberry (eds). *Ferrets, Rabbits, and Rodents: Clinical Medicine and Surgery*. W.B. Saunders, Philadelphia, pp. 392–403.

Williams, B.H. (1996) Pathology of the domestic ferret. Proceedings of a C.L. Davis Foundation European Symposium.

Chapter 12

Besch-Williford, C.L. (1987) Biology and medicine of the ferret. *Veterinary Clinics of North America: Small Animal Practice*, **17**, pp. 1155–83.

Burke, T.J. (1988) Common diseases and medical management of ferrets. In: E.R. Jacobson and G.V. Kollias (eds). *Exotic Animals*. Churchill Livingstone, Edinburgh, pp. 247–60.

Erdman, S.E., Li, X. and Fox, J.G. (1998) Haematopoietic diseases. In: J.G. Fox (ed.). *Biology and Diseases of the Ferret*. 2nd edn. Williams and Wilkins, Baltimore, pp. 231–46.

Fox, J.G. (1998) Parasitic diseases. In: J.G. Fox (ed.). *Biology and Diseases of the Ferret*. 2nd edn. Williams and Wilkins, Baltimore, pp. 375–91.

Fox, J.G. (1998) Other systemic diseases. In: J.G. Fox (ed.). *Biology and Diseases of the Ferret*. 2nd edn. Williams and Wilkins, Baltimore, pp. 307–20.

Randolph, R.W. (1989) Medical and surgical care in the pet ferret. In: R.W. Kirk (ed.). *Current Veterinary Therapy X*. W.B. Saunders, Philadelphia, pp. 765–75.

Rosenthal, K. (1994) Ferrets. *Veterinary Clinics of North America: Small Animal Practice*, **24**, pp. 1–23.

Stamoulis, M.E. and Miller, M.S. (1997) Cardiac diseases. In: E.V. Hillyer and K.E. Quesenberry (eds). *Ferrets, Rabbits, and Rodents: Clinical Medicine and Surgery*. W.B. Saunders, Philadelphia, pp. 63–70.

Williams, B.H. (1996) Pathology of the domestic ferret. Proceedings of a C.L. Davis Foundation European Symposium.

Chapter 13

Bell, J.A. (1997) Periparturient and neonatal diseases. In: E.V. Hillyer and K.E. Quesenberry (eds). *Ferrets, Rabbits, and Rodents: Clinical Medicine and Surgery.* W.B. Saunders, Philadelphia, pp. 53–62.

Bernard, S.L., Gorham, J.R. and Ryland, R.M. (1984) Biology and diseases of ferrets: IV–VI diseases. In: J.G. Fox, B.J. Cohen and F.M. Loew (eds). *Laboratory Animal Medicine.* Academic Press, Orlando, pp. 389–97.

Brown, S.A. (1997) Neoplasia. In: E.V. Hillyer and K.E. Quesenberry (eds). *Ferrets, Rabbits, and Rodents: Clinical Medicine and Surgery.* W.B. Saunders, Philadelphia, pp. 99–114.

Fox, J.G., Pearson, R.C. and Bell, J.A. (1998) Diseases of the genitourinary system. In: J.G. Fox (ed.). *Biology and Diseases of the Ferret.* 2nd edn. Williams and Wilkins, Baltimore, pp. 247–72.

Hillyer, E.V. (1997) Urogenital diseases. In: E.V. Hillyer and K.E. Quesenberry (eds). *Ferrets, Rabbits, and Rodents: Clinical Medicine and Surgery.* W.B. Saunders, Philadelphia, pp. 44–52.

Oxenham, M. (1991) Ferrets. In: P.H. Beynon and J.E. Cooper (eds). *Manual of Exotic Pets.* British Small Animal Veterinary Association, Cheltenham, pp. 97–109.

Rosenthal, K. (1994) Ferrets. *Veterinary Clinics of North America: Small Animal Practice,* **24**, pp. 1–23.

Williams, B.H. (1996) Pathology of the domestic ferret. Proceedings of a C.L. Davis Foundation European Symposium.

Wolvekamp, P. (1998) Radiography of small mammals: techniques and interpretation. Paper given at BSAVA Congress, Birmingham, UK.

Chapter 14

Besch-Williford, C.L. (1987) Biology and medicine of the ferret. *Veterinary Clinics of North America: Small Animal Practice,* **17**, pp. 1155–83.

Brooks, H.V., Rammell, C.G., Hoogenboom, J.J.L. and Taylor, D.E.S. (1985) Observations on an outbreak of nutritional steatitis (yellow fat disease) in fitch (*Mustela putorius furo*). *New Zealand Veterinary Journal*, **33**, pp. 141–5.

Fox, J.G. and McLain, D.E. (1998) Nutrition. In: J.G. Fox (ed.). *Biology and Diseases of the Ferret*. 2nd edn. Williams and Wilkins, Baltimore, pp. 149–72.

Oxenham, M. (1991) Ferrets. In: P.H. Beynon and J.E. Cooper (eds). *Manual of Exotic Pets*. British Small Animal Veterinary Association, Cheltenham, pp. 97–109.

Porter, V. and Brown, N. (1997) *The Complete Book of Ferrets*. D & M Publications, Bedford.

Straube, E.F. and Walden, N.B. (1981) Zinc poisoning in ferrets (*Mustela putorius furo*). *Laboratory Animals*, **15**, pp. 45–7.

Chapter 15

Batchelder, M.A., Erdman, S.E., Li, X. and Fox, J.G. (1996) Cluster of cases of juvenile mediastinal lymphoma in a ferret colony. *Laboratory Animal Science*, **46**, pp. 271–4.

Brown, S.A. (1997) Neoplasia. In: E.V. Hillyer and K.E. Quesenberry (eds). *Ferrets, Rabbits, and Rodents: Clinical Medicine and Surgery*. W.B. Saunders, Philadelphia, pp. 99–114.

Brown, S.A. (1998) Diagnosis and management of neoplastic disease in ferrets. Paper given at BSAVA Congress, Birmingham, UK.

Dillberger, J.E. and Altman, N.H. (1989) Neoplasia in ferrets: eleven cases with a review. *Journal of Comparative Pathology*, **100**, pp. 161–76.

Erdman, S.E., Brown, S.A., Kawasaki, T.A., Moore, F.M., Li, X. and Fox, J.G. (1996) Clinical and pathological findings in ferrets with lymphoma: 60 cases (1982–1994). *Journal of the American Veterinary Medical Association*, **208**, pp. 1285–9.

Erdman, S.E., Li, X. and Fox, J.G. (1998) Haematopoietic diseases. In: J.G. Fox (ed.). *Biology and Diseases of the Ferret*. 2nd edn. Williams and Wilkins, Baltimore, pp. 231–46.

Li, X. and Fox, J.G. (1998) Neoplastic diseases. In: J.G. Fox (ed.). *Biology and Diseases of the Ferret*. 2nd edn. Williams and Wilkins, Baltimore, pp. 405–47.

Li, X., Fox, J.G. and Erdman, S.E. (1996) Multiple splenic myelolipomas in a ferret (*Mustela putorius furo*). *Laboratory Animal Science*, **46**, pp. 101–3.

Rosenthal, K. (1994) Ferrets. *Veterinary Clinics of North America: Small Animal Practice*, **24**, pp. 1–23.

Rudmann, D.G., White, M.R. and Murphey, J.B. (1994) Complex ceruminous gland adenocarcinoma in a brown footed ferret (*Mustela putorius furo*). *Laboratory Animal Science*, **44**, pp. 637–8.

Sleeman, Y.M., Clyde, V.L. and Brenneman, K.A. (1996) Granular cell tumour in the central nervous system of a ferret (*Mustela putorius furo*). *Veterinary Record*, **138**, pp. 65–6.

Taylor, T.G. and Carpenter, J.L. (1995) Thymoma in two ferrets. *Laboratory Animal Science*, **45**, pp. 363–5.

Williams, B.H. (1996) Pathology of the domestic ferret. Proceedings of a C.L. Davis Foundation European Symposium.

SECTION 3
APPROACH TO CLINICAL
EXAMINATION AND
DIAGNOSIS

16 CLINICAL EXAMINATION OF THE FERRET

Many veterinary practitioners will be unused to ferrets and may be unsure how to approach them in the consulting room. Stories of painful ferret bites and the use of ferrets for rabbiting may lead to anxiety on the part of the clinician, making a ferret consultation a stressful experience. These anxieties however are for the most part unfounded, and the examination and treatment of pet ferrets should be no more difficult than for cats or dogs. The use of diagnostic tools such as radiography and clinical pathology are as useful in ferrets as in other species, and treatments can often follow guidelines for cats and dogs.

Ferrets are stoic animals and tend to mask clinical signs. Often, ferret owners will consult other ferret owners about their animals before coming to the veterinarian, so they may be very ill when first presented for examination. Be sure to take a full history from the owner, noting particularly the vaccination status of the animal and any other animals in the household.

Handling

The important rules when handling ferrets are:

(1)   Be positive, calm and confident;
(2)   Know what you are doing;
(3)   Keep movements smooth and decisive; and
(4)   Use your voice as well as your hands.

Ferrets are usually friendly, docile creatures which will rarely bite, particularly if handled from an early age, although particular care must be taken with nursing jills and animals which are not used to being handled, as these may be more prone to aggression. Their eyesight is relatively poor, so their reactions are reflex and instant. A hesitant approaching finger will be mistaken for a prey object and may be bitten, so it is important that all movements are direct and deliberate. Talk to the animal as you approach him so he knows you are there, and reward his good behaviour with a friendly rub after the examination. Most ferrets will also appreciate being given a treat such as a lick of Nutri-plus Gel (Virbac).

Normally, only minimal restraint will be required in order to perform a clinical examination. Allow the ferret to run free on the surface of the consulting table for a few minutes after the owner has removed him from the transport box, so that he may explore and become accustomed to the new surroundings. It is unlikely that a ferret will jump or fall from the edge of the table, and giving him time to calm down reduces the risk of being bitten or of having him express his anal glands. Take this time to observe the animal's general demeanour and behaviour. Often ferrets will sleep during the day and may need to be woken up for the examination, but once awakened they should soon become alert, exploring the environment vigorously. Lethargy or non-responsiveness are signs of ill health.

Once the animal appears to be calm, distract him by waving a cloth or sleeve in front of his nose with one hand, then grasp the animal firmly and deliberately with the other hand, either over the shoulders or alternatively with thumb and forefinger encircling the neck with the other fingers under the forelimbs. This way, the animal is not interested in the hand which is approaching from above to pick him up and will not try to bite it (see Figure 16.1). It is normal for the animal to wriggle initially while it is being held. Lift the animal up and support the hind quarters with the other hand. Ferrets normally react to being picked up in this manner by relaxing and becoming immobile. If extra restraint is required, placing a little pressure over the animal's elbows will cause the forefeet to cross over giving added

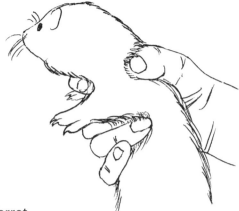

Figure 16.1   Handling the ferret.

security against bites and scratches. Very rarely, an aggressive ferret may need to be scruffed, although this may be interpreted by adult ferrets as either an aggressive encounter or a courtship ritual, which may produce an unexpected reaction. Leather gloves may be needed, but these need to be very thick otherwise the ferret will bite through them, and so should only be used in exceptional circumstances. Ferrets should never be lifted by the tail.

Ferrets have a tenacious grip: ferret bites can easily penetrate down to the bone, and removing an animal from a finger can be a difficult task. If a ferret's feet are not touching the floor, it will hang on with its teeth despite all attempts to disengage it. If this occurs, place the animal's feet onto a solid surface before attempting to prise the jaws apart. Very rarely if this fails, applying some isopropyl alcohol to the animal's gum or placing the animal's head under cold running water will encourage them to let go.

When angry or frightened, ferrets will hiss or scream, which gives the handler warning that the animal may be difficult to handle. Such animals may need to be sedated for examination.

Clinical examination

In order to ensure that all areas are examined, it is sensible to begin at the head end and work backwards systematically. However, ferrets will object strongly to having their rectal temperature taken and may struggle violently, and a measurement taken at the start of the consultation is less likely to be artificially elevated by the stress of the consultation than one taken at the end. It is a good idea to use a plastic digital thermometer which is unlikely to break, rather than a glass one.

Note the condition of the eyes, nose, and ears, and look for facial symmetry. Check for evidence of cataracts or corneal drying, ensure the mucous membranes are moist, look for evidence of *Otodectes cynotis* in the ears (normally there is very little earwax), and lift the upper lip to examine the teeth and gingiva and to assess capillary refill time.

Assess the animal's hydration status by checking for skin turgor. Palpate the lymph nodes in the submandibular, axillary, popliteal and inguinal regions for signs of enlargement or asymmetry. In fat animals, they may appear enlarged due to fat deposition, so overall body condition and the time of year need to be taken into account when assessing the significance of any enlarged lymph nodes.

Check the feet for the length of the claws and for any pododermatitis, which may occur if the animal is kept in damp conditions. Ferrets' claws are non-retractile. Working ferrets may need to keep their claws long. To clip the nails, try applying some Nutri-plus Gel (Virbac) to the abdomen. The animal will lick the gel and stick its legs in the air, making access to the nails easy.

Auscultate the chest, listening for cardiac arrhythmias or murmurs, and any abnormal lung sounds. The heart lies between the sixth and eighth ribs, so auscultation is performed in a more caudal location to other species. Ferrets have a high heart rate (180–250 bpm), and may have a pronounced sinus arrhythmia. Cardiomyopathies are common in older ferrets, and any abnormality is worthy of investigation. Lung sounds should be minimal: any changes are likely to be subtle so the examination should be carried out in a quiet environment.

The abdomen can be examined with the animal lifted wholly or partly off the table. In a relaxed animal, the abdominal organs can be palpated readily, and holding the animal in a semi-vertical position allows the cranial abdominal organs to become more accessible. Alternatively, hold the animal around the shoulders, and turn him onto his back, supporting it with your forearm with his hindfeet tucked beneath your upper arm. Palpate the abdomen gently in order not to cause any damage, particularly if there is a suspicion of intestinal foreign body. Check for gas accumulations or irregular masses in the stomach area. It is quite common for the spleen to be enlarged, but this is often insignificant and should be interpreted in the light of any other abnormal findings. Feel for the liver, kidneys, intestines and urinary bladder as with other animals, to detect enlargements or irregularities.

Check the perineal area for evidence of abnormal discharges, diarrhoea, mucus or blood. In a female, ascertain the reproductive status of the animal and examine the vulva. An enlarged vulva in a spayed female is usually consistent with a functional adrenal tumour or an ovarian remnant. In an intact female determine how long the animal has been in oestrus and check the mucous membranes for evidence of petechiae, which may indicate bone marrow depression due to hyperoestrogenism. In males, the testicles descend into the scrotal area only between December and September, when they are easily palpable. Check for symmetry and texture: they should have the consistency of small ripe tomatoes.

Check through the hair coat for evidence of parasites, skin tumours or alopecia. Hair loss from the tail tip is a common and frequently incidental finding, and breeding animals often exhibit partial alopecia which resolves during the quiescent period. Bilaterally symmetrical alopecia which is not seasonal or which progresses cranially may be an indication of an underlying hormonal imbalance such as adrenal-related endocrinopathy.

Often, sufficient information will be available from the clinical examination to make a diagnosis and begin treatment. If not, further work up will be required. This may include diagnostic imaging including radiography, and the taking of blood or other samples (see Chapter 17).

Radiography

The small size and constant activity of ferrets means that it is difficult to position them accurately for radiography without sedation or general anaesthesia. Restraint can be achieved by placing the animal in a tube, but positioning is poor and interpretation of the films becomes difficult. Manual restraint is not recommended for health and safety reasons. The best diagnostic information comes from exact positioning, and this can be achieved by placing the anaesthetised or sedated animal on a perspex plate and securing it with radiolucent masking tape. The plate can then be placed over the x-ray cassette. Alternatively, small foam rubber wedges or cradles can be used. Although the small size of ferrets means a powerful X-ray machine is not essential, a high mA capacity allows for short exposure times, minimising movement blur. Most exposures can be taken at 50 kV, altering the mAs as required. See Plates 17 and 18 for normal lateral and dorso-ventral radiographs.

Radiological changes are likely to be very subtle, so it is important to obtain high quality, detailed radiographs. A high mA allows high definition, slow speed film–screen combinations or non-screen film to be used. Detail can also be enhanced by collimating the x-ray beam, and reducing scatter as much as possible. Placing a lead sheet over the cassette with a window beneath the area of interest will help to reduce scatter, and allow several images to be recorded on one plate.

For limbs, it is best to use non-screen film in order to gain a sufficiently detailed image. For other areas, using a high mA and short exposure time with a slow speed film, or a slow rare earth screen and film combination, will allow shorter exposure times to keep movement blur to a minimum, while maintaining a high definition image.

When taking thoracic radiographs, it is important to remember that ferrets have a very long tubular body, and the exposed area must include the thoracic inlet and the last rib in order to cover the entire lung field. The cone shaped heart extends approximately from the sixth to eighth rib, with the apex to the left of the midline.

Quantities of fat may be deposited in the ligament which joins the heart to the sternum, and on lateral radiography the heart shadow appears to be raised above the sternum. Loss of this space can be an indicator of cardiac enlargement.

Abdominal radiographs can be taken and interpreted as for cats or dogs. Centre the beam between the last rib and wing of the ilium and extend the animal's legs caudally.

To get the best out of a film, it is essential to maintain the quality of processing, to ensure that the films are fully developed and there is sufficient contrast. Automatic processors will give uniformly developed films, and aid in interpretation.

Post mortem examination

It is likely that some animals will succumb without a diagnosis having been made, whatever treatment is given, and a thorough post mortem examination may be useful in determining the cause of death. This should involve a thorough examination of the whole carcase, and each organ should be removed and inspected. It is useful to have a cork board for pinning the carcase and some instruments set aside specifically for post mortem examinations.

Procedure

(1)   Weigh the animal and examine the external appearance of the carcase. Make a note of the body condition, and examine all external orifices for any abnormalities or discharges. Examine the feet, tail and skin for any lesions and note any evidence of vomiting, diarrhoea or dehydration. In the female, examine the vulva for swelling, and look for petechial haemorrhages on the mucous membrane. Take samples of the skin and hair if there are any abnormalities.

(2)   Lay the animal out on its back and pin the feet to the board if necessary to support the carcase. Swab the ventral surface liberally with disinfectant to reduce bacterial contamination and prevent pollution of the area with dander and fur.

(3) Make a midline skin incision from mandible to pubis and reflect the skin away from the midline. Remove the muscles over the thorax and open the chest cavity by holding the xiphisternum and cutting through the costochondral junctions on each side. Reflect the sternum and ribs anteriorly to expose the underlying viscera. Observe the thoracic viscera *in situ*, noting any abnormalities such as discoloration in the lungs, or fluid in the pleural cavity or pericardium. Open the trachea and note any inflammation or fluid inside.

(4) Open the abdominal wall with a straight midline incision and reflect the wall sideways. Again, look at the organs *in situ* and note any obvious changes such as liver abscessation or fluid in the peritoneal cavity.

(5) Grasp the trachea and oesophagus, cut across and lift upwards to remove the heart and lungs, easing away any dorsal connections. Cut across the oesophagus as it passes through the diaphragm and remove the thoracic viscera for a more thorough examination on a separate tray. Look for areas of discoloration, altered texture, adhesions or other abnormalities. Open the length of the trachea, oesophagus, and bronchi. Cut through the lung lobes and squeeze gently to see if there is any fluid present in the lung parenchyma. Open the heart by incising from the apex of the left ventricle up into the left atrium and into the aorta, and from the apex of the right ventricle up into the right atrium and into the pulmonary artery. This method ensures that the heart valves and endocardium can be examined undamaged by the dissection.

(6) Examine the intestinal tract carefully noting such facts as whether the stomach is full or empty, whether the gut is full of gas, fluid or solid matter or any areas of inflammation. Remove the intestinal tract and examine the mesenteric lymph nodes and the inside surface of the stomach and intestines. Remember the small and large intestines are difficult to distinguish.

(7) Cut around the dorsal surface of the liver to remove it and cut

through the lobes. Examine the cut surface for variations in the normal architecture.

(8) Examine the uro-genital tract. Incise the kidneys longitudinally and inspect the internal structure. Peel off the capsule.

(9) The eviscerated carcase should then be examined for any other abnormalities such as enlarged joints or lymph nodes. If the history indicates it, the head can be removed to take out the brain for detailed inspection.

Samples of diseased tissues may be sent to a laboratory for further investigation. It is often of use to take samples of lung, liver and intestines for routine bacteriological examination, even if there are no obvious abnormalities. For example, bacterial septicaemia may result in death with few overt signs, but culture of the liver would reveal the cause of death. Histological examination of diseased tissues may also be of particular value.

A post mortem examination to determine the cause of death may seem to be unnecessarily complex for a single animal, but if the owner has several animals, a thorough examination of any animals which die unexpectedly could prove invaluable in preventing an epidemic of any potentially fatal diseases.

17 SAMPLE COLLECTION AND DRUG ADMINISTRATION

Sample collection

Blood

Blood may be collected relatively easily from conscious animals if they are used to being handled, but if not then sedation or anaesthesia may be required. Choose sedatives with care, since some agents interfere with haematology. Isoflurane anaesthesia produces a fall in packed cell volume, haemoglobin level and red cell count, possibly due to sequestering of cells in the spleen. The author has successfully used combinations of midazolam and ketamine to provide sedation for blood sampling.

Blood may be collected from a number of sites, depending on the required volume. As with any animal, the sample taken must be sufficiently large for the required tests to be performed, without causing any disturbance to the animal's physiology. To avoid any problems, a single sample should be a maximum of 10% of the animal's total blood volume, and if serial samples are to be taken, not more than 15% of blood volume should be taken in a 28 day period. The total blood volume is approximately 70 ml/kg body weight, so for an average female weighing 750 g a suitable volume for a single sample would be 5 ml, and for a male of 1.5 kg up to 10 ml can be taken.

A small sample may be collected from conscious animals by clipping a toenail and allowing blood to be drawn into a capillary tube or 'Microvette'® (Sarstedt). These can be obtained coated with various anticoagulants. This method can be used for collecting samples for measurement of the PCV or for Aleutian disease virus testing.

Larger samples can be obtained by peripheral venepuncture. In conscious restrained ferrets, samples can be obtained using the ventral tail artery or veins. With the animal held on its back by an assistant, shave the hair from the ventral aspect of the proximal tail. The tail appears to have a flattened area on the ventral side for the proximal 4–5 cm, and this represents the ventral concavity of the caudal vertebrae. The artery lies 2–3 mm beneath the surface of the skin and is flanked by two smaller veins. Use a 21G or 23G needle or winged infusion set for venepuncture. Swab the skin with 70% ethanol, then hold the tail with the free hand and insert the needle at a shallow angle towards the body in the midline, 3–4 cm from the base of the tail. As the needle enters the vessel, blood will appear in the hub of the needle and gentle suction will allow 0.5–1.0 ml of blood to be withdrawn from the vein, or 3–5 ml from the artery. Apply pressure for 1–2 minutes after removal of the needle to prevent haematoma formation.

Jugular venepuncture may be carried out in friendly animals by wrapping them firmly in a towel making sure the fore limbs are restrained. Alternatively the animal may be sedated or anaesthetised. The animal is held on its back with the neck extended by an assistant: this can be facilitated by placing some pleasant foodstuff such as Marmite or Nutri-plus gel (Virbac) on the animal's nose, so the animal stretches his head back trying to reach it. Stand with the animal's head towards you. Shave the ventral aspect of the neck and swab it with alcohol, place a hand beneath the neck to support it, and raise the jugular vein by applying pressure at the thoracic inlet. Insert a 21G or 23G 25mm (1 inch) needle at a shallow angle through the skin and into the vein pointing towards the heart. This can be facilitated by bending the needle up slightly to an angle of approximately 30° (see Figure 17.1). It is sometimes easier to put the needle through the skin slightly lateral to the vein, then redirect it into the vein once through the skin. A 'pop' may be felt as the needle enters the vein. Jugular venepuncture is most successful if carried

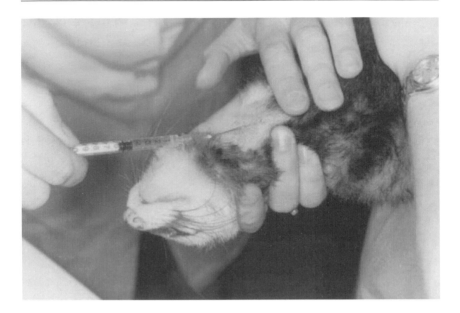

Figure 17.1 Jugular venepuncture.

out near the thoracic inlet where the jugular vein joins the anterior vena cava.

The lateral saphenous vein can be cannulated to allow repeated blood sampling or intravenous administration. The vein can be found on the lateral surface of the distal hind leg. In the conscious restrained or sedated animal, shave the area overlying the vein: a tourniquet may be used above the stifle to raise the vein. After nicking the skin with a needle or scalpel blade, insert a 24G 19 mm ($\frac{3}{4}$ inch) over the needle cannula and tape it in place. If it is to be maintained for long periods, it should be flushed frequently with sterile (heparinised) saline and covered with soft bandage to prevent interference by the animal.

Samples may be collected into anticoagulants for haematological, serological or biochemical examination. Ferrets have a high packed cell volume and a slow erythrocyte sedimentation rate, so when centrifuging ferret blood in order to collect serum or plasma or for measurement of the PCV, the blood must be spun for 20% longer than other blood samples, and three times the required plasma volume must be collected. Normal values for haematology and biochemistry may be found in Section 4, Tables 20.2 and 20.3.

Urine/faeces

Ferrets are clean animals and will tend to urinate and defaecate in one area of the cage. Since the gut transit time is short, faeces is passed quite frequently and fresh samples can easily be collected from the latrine area.

Urine may be collected as it is voided naturally by housing the animal temporarily in a cage with a grid floor and collecting it from a tray placed beneath the cage. Gentle manual expression of the bladder is also possible.

Sterile samples may be collected by cystocentesis provided the bladder is full. The bladder wall is muscular and can easily be lacerated in conscious animals, so always sedate or anaesthetise the animal for this procedure. The method is similar for that used in cats or dogs. Clip and prepare the caudal abdomen as for surgery, palpate and immobilise the bladder with one hand, and use a 25G 16 mm ($\frac{5}{8}$ inch) needle to withdraw urine directly from the bladder with the other.

Urethral catheterisation of the bladder is difficult in ferrets, but may be necessary for the collection of sterile urine samples or for contrast radiography. It can be achieved in anaesthetised animals as follows. For females, position them in ventral recumbency with the hind quarters elevated, and disinfect the skin around the vulva with a suitable agent such as chlorhexidine solution. The urethral opening can be located using a speculum on the floor of the vestibule approximately 1 cm anterior to the clitoral fossa. A lubricated 3 or 3.5 French gauge rubber urinary catheter with a wire stylet may then be passed gently through the urethra into the bladder. For males, place the animal in dorsal recumbency, exteriorise the penis and clean the skin as above. A 3 or 3.5 FG soft rubber catheter without a stylet can then be passed into the urethral opening. Tom cat catheters are not suitable since they tend to be too stiff and will not easily pass through the os penis and around the ischial arch.

Normal values for urinalysis can be found in Section 4, Table 20.4.

Skin and hair samples

Samples of hair may be plucked from the edges of skin lesions for the diagnosis of dermatophytoses, and skin scrapings can be useful for the diagnosis of external parasites. However, it is often more valuable to perform biopsies of skin lesions under anaesthesia. Skin neoplasms are not uncommon, so fine needle aspirates should be taken from any nodules to ascertain if neoplastic cells are present. If so, an excisional biopsy should be performed.

Cytology and microbiology

Impression smears and needle aspirates are easy to perform and can provide much diagnostic information. Place a clean glass slide on the cut surface of the affected tissue or apply aspirated material to the slide. Take care when aspirating lymph nodes percutaneously however, since ferrets have perinodal fat pads and obtaining samples from the actual node can be difficult. Excisional biopsies may be better for lymph nodes.

Microbiological examination can be performed on needle aspirates, or on swabs taken from the lesion placed into an appropriate transport medium. It is helpful to determine the requirements of the laboratory before taking samples. Wait for about one hour after taking swabs for the bacteria to colonise the swab before refrigeration. When taking swabs from abscesses, take the sample from the wall of the lesion, not the pus from the centre which is likely to be sterile.

Bone marrow

A bone marrow sample may be necessary for the correct diagnosis of non-regenerative anaemias and other disorders of blood cells. Bone marrow aspirates may be taken from the proximal femur in anaesthetised ferrets. Place the animal in lateral recumbency and clip and prepare the skin overlying the proximal femur for surgery. Make a stab incision in the skin over the femur medial to the greater trochanter, and insert a 20G 40 mm (1.5 inch) spinal needle through the incision and into the bone using a rotating action, pointing towards the foot. Once in the marrow cavity, remove the stylet from the needle and apply a syringe. Vigorous suction should be applied until marrow fluid appears in the syringe, then suction should cease to prevent contamination of the sample with blood. Apply the material obtained to several slides immediately, and prepare and stain as for other species.

This technique for penetration of bone marrow may also be used if it is necessary to administer fluids by the intraosseous route.

Semen

Samples of semen may be collected by electroejaculation in anaesthetised animals. Inhalation anaesthetics, diazepam and ace-promazine all cause relaxation of the bladder musculature and may result in contamination of the sample with urine. This is less of a problem when using medetomidine or xylazine and ketamine. Carnivore semen is sensitive to handling, and care must be taken with the processing method to ensure sperm viability. The semen should be collected into a warmed glass or plastic collection vessel to prevent cold shock to the sperm.

A 6 mm probe with longitudinal electrodes is best. The lubricated probe is inserted into the rectum and positioned over the accessory sex glands. Moving the probe in a cranio-caudal direction over these glands during electroejaculation can enhance the volume of ejaculate.

A total of 80 stimulations given in three series is usually successful. Begin each stimulation with the voltage at zero, build up to the required level over one second, hold for two to three seconds, then finish abruptly. Rest for three seconds between stimulations, and for two to three minutes between series. Series one consists of ten stimulations at 4 V, ten at 5 V and ten at 6 V. Series two consists of ten stimulations at 5 V, ten at 6 V and ten at 7 V, and series three consists of ten at 6 V, and ten at 7 V.

The normal volume which can be collected is 0.05 ± 0.01 ml, containing approximately 706×10^6 spermatozoa per ml. Approximately 67% should be normal, with 80% motility.

Drug administration

Oral administration

Drugs are most easily given orally in liquid form or suspension, although pills may be administered in compliant animals. Hold the animal by the neck in dorsal recumbency, and use a syringe to place the medication onto the back of the tongue. A stomach tube may also be passed this way. Palatable medicaments may be given in the feed.

Subcutaneous administration

Subcutaneous injections should be given between the shoulder blades, or in the scruff of the neck. The skin is very tough here, and a 23G 25 mm (1 inch) needle may be required to penetrate the skin. Ferrets seem to find subcutaneous injections uncomfortable, and good restraint is required to prevent the handler from being bitten.

Intramuscular administration

Intramuscular injections may be given into the quadriceps muscle on the front of the thigh, or the hamstrings on the caudal thigh. The animal is restrained by an assistant and the muscle located and immobilised with one hand while the injection is given with the other.

Intravenous administration

Intravenous injections may be given into the jugular, lateral saphenous, or tail vein using methods as described above, using a needle and syringe or winged infusion set. Alternatively, the cephalic vein may be used. This can be found by shaving the dorsal surface of the antebrachium and raising the vein near the elbow as for cats and dogs. It is often better to raise the vein using a tourniquet rather than a hand, since the foreleg is short. A 27G 1.2 mm needle will easily enter the vein, or a 24G 19 mm ($\frac{3}{4}$ inch) over-the-needle cannula can be used. In order to prevent the cannula from buckling, the tough skin overlying the vein may be nicked using a needle or scalpel blade. The cannula can then be passed easily into the vein and secured using adhesive tape.

Other

Intraosseous administration of blood or fluids may be necessary in severely ill animals. Access to the marrow cavity in the proximal femur may be gained as described above on page 154 for bone marrow collection.

18 SEDATION, ANAESTHESIA AND ANALGESIA

In clinical veterinary practice, it is not uncommon to find that the mortality rate under general anaesthesia for small mammals such as ferrets is higher than that found for cats and dogs. There are several possible reasons for this. Practitioners may be unfamiliar with the species, they may have little knowledge of the particular considerations which need to be given to these animals during anaesthesia and surgery, and the health of the animal prior to anaesthesia may be poor. As with any surgical procedure involving anaesthesia, careful planning and preparation will reduce any risks.

Pre-anaesthetic considerations

Check the health of the animal very carefully in the pre-operative consultation, paying particular attention to the cardiovascular and respiratory systems, and obtain an accurate weight. The pre-operative check may include taking a sample of blood for complete haematology and assessment of hepatic and renal function. Any disturbance to the animal's health may reduce the delivery of oxygen to the tissues, and in this case surgery should be delayed until the animal is well, particularly with an elective procedure.

Animals which are stressed by transport and poor handling in the immediate pre-anaesthetic period will have high circulating catecholamine levels. This will increase the dose of anaesthetic required for induction, increasing any side effects, and these animals will be more prone to developing potentially fatal cardiac arrhythmias during the operation. Ensure the animal is calm before attempting to anaesthetise it, which may require the administration of a sedative, and is always handled properly.

Ferrets will vomit readily, and should be fasted for a period prior to anaesthesia. Due to the short gut transit time, this period need not exceed four to six hours. Longer periods of fasting may lead to hypoglycaemia, increasing the risks associated with anaesthesia. Free access to water should be given until immediately prior to the induction of anaesthesia.

Premedication may be given to allay fear and anxiety, to smooth induction and reduce the dose of induction agent required, to provide post-operative analgesia, to smooth recovery, or to dry bronchial secretions. Intramuscular or subcutaneous injections of a suitable premed can be given readily to most conscious restrained ferrets. Combinations of sedatives with or without analgesics and drying agents can be given, depending on the type of procedure and the temperament of the animal. For example, for short, non-painful procedures such as radiography or nail clipping, premedication with diazepam may be sufficient. For a major surgical procedure such as ovariohysterectomy, a combination including sedative, analgesic and drying agent may be required. Since the airways are small and easily become blocked with mucus, drying agents should be given before induction of general anaesthesia. Suggested doses of sedatives and premedicants are given in Table 18.1.

General anaesthesia

Following a suitable premedicant, or even omitting this step with very friendly ferrets, general anaesthesia may be induced by the intravenous administration of anaesthetic into the cephalic vein on the forelimb. Alternatively, intramuscular administration of inject-able agents will result in the induction of anaesthesia within a few minutes in most animals. Injectable agents should be dosed by weight, but account should be taken of the time of year, since ferrets accumulate fat in the winter and may require relatively more anaesthetic during this period.

Table 18.1 Suggested sedatives and premedicants for ferrets.

Drug	Dose	Comments
Midazolam with ketamine	0.2 mg/kg with 10 mg/kg	Mix in same syringe, administer i.m. Good short term sedation with relaxation suitable for minor procedures such as radiography.
Medetomidine	100 μg/kg i.v., i.m. or s.c.	Can reverse with atipamezole. Useful for minor non-painful procedures or premedication.
Diazepam or midazolam	2 mg/kg i.m.	Reduces anxiety and produces relaxation.
Xylazine	1 mg/kg i.v., i.m. or s.c.	Hypotensive.
Ketamine	20–30 mg/kg i.m.	Poor muscle relaxation if used alone.
Acepromazine	0.2–0.5 mg/kg s.c. or i.m.	Hypotensive.
Fentanyl/fluanisone	0.5 ml/kg i.m.	Neuroleptanalgesia with poor muscle relaxation.
Atropine	0.05 mg/kg s.c.	Dries airway secretions.

Volatile anaesthetics are very useful for both induction and maintenance of anaesthesia, and can be used following induction with injectable agents. Suitably restrained or premedicated animals can be induced using isoflurane or halothane with oxygen via a face mask or an induction chamber: do not use the same chamber that is used for rodents, since the smell of the ferret will cause distress to any rodents placed in the chamber subsequently. Once the animal is immobile and relaxed, anaesthesia can be maintained using a low resistance circuit, such as a T-piece, and a face mask. Nitrous oxide may be added to the inspired gas mixture to provide additional analgesia. Use it 60:40 or 50:50 with oxygen. Table 18.2 gives recommended induction and maintenance concentrations for volatile agents. Endotracheal intubation is recommended for longer procedures. A modified urinary catheter may make a suitable endotracheal tube if a paediatric ET tube is too large: 2.5–4 mm tubes are usually used. Place the animal in sternal recumbency and have an assistant bend the head upwards as far as possible by placing thumb and forefinger in the corners of the mouth. Pull the

Table 18.2   Use of volatile agents in ferrets.

Volatile agent	Induction concentration	Maintenance concentration
Isoflurane	3–4%	1.5–3%
Halothane	2–4%	0.8–2%

tongue forwards and over the lower incisors to depress the mandible. Advance the lubricated tube into the mouth: a laryngoscope may help to visualise the larynx, and slide the tube gently through the glottis.

A recommended method for general anaesthesia is to use medetomidine with ketamine for induction, transferring to isoflurane with oxygen and nitrous oxide for maintenance. Once the animal is connected to the isoflurane, the medetomidine can be reversed with atipamezole.

Suitable combinations of injectable drugs for anaesthesia with or without premedication are given in Table 18.3.

Anaesthetic management

During general anaesthesia it is important to monitor the animal's physiological stability. Check the animal's respiration and cardiovascular system every few minutes. Always administer oxygen, even if using an injectable agent, since animals may be in poor health and many anaesthetics cause respiratory depression. Respiratory failure is a common cause of anaesthetic emergencies in ferrets.

Ensure the animal is able to maintain its body temperature. Hypothermia is common due to the high metabolic rate and high surface area to volume ratio. Keep the animal warm throughout the procedure by wrapping it up and providing supplementary heating if necessary. The depth of anaesthesia can be determined by checking for the absence of somatic reflexes such as the pedal withdrawal reflex, assessing the degree of muscle tone, and observing any changes in the heart and respiratory rates in response to surgical stimulation.

Table 18.3 Suitable agents for general anaesthesia in the ferret.

Drug	Dose	Comments
Medetomidine with ketamine	100–120 µg/kg with 8–10 mg/kg	Mix in same syringe, administer i.m. Surgical anaesthesia for 20–30 minutes. Can reverse with atipamezole, 0.25–0.5 mg/kg i.m. Care in pregnant animals: potentially abortifacient.
Xylazine with ketamine	1–4 mg/kg with 25 mg/kg i.m.	As above but with more respiratory depression.
Alphaxalone/ alphadolone	12 mg/kg i.v., 10–15 mg/kg i.m.	Short anaesthesia with good relaxation. Some respiratory depression. Incremental doses 6–8 mg/kg i.v. for prolonged anaesthesia.
Ketamine with diazepam	25 mg/kg with 2 mg/kg i.m.	Surgical anaesthesia for approx 30 minutes. Less respiratory depression than with α_2 agonists.
Ketamine with acepromazine	25 mg/kg with 0.25 mg/kg i.m.	As above.
Propofol	10 mg/kg i.v.	Can be used for total intravenous anaesthesia.

Post-operative care and analgesia

Following surgery it is important to continue monitoring the animal's vital signs, and keep the body temperature up until the animal has fully regained consciousness. It is also important to maintain the animal's fluid balance during and after general anaesthesia to prevent dehydration and hypovolaemia. The daily fluid requirement is approximately 75–100 ml/kg, and in addition to this the clinician must account for any blood or fluid loss during surgery, and pre-existing dehydration, or losses due to vomiting etc. Fluids can be given intravenously into the cephalic or lateral saphenous veins. Calculate the fluid deficit, and administer warmed saline, Hartmann's solution or dextrose saline by slow intravenous infusion so as not to overload the lungs. If venous access is not possible, fluid may be given subcutaneously in several sites. If the animal is in extremis, blood or fluid may be given directly into the bone marrow (see page 154).

Blood transfusions may be necessary if there has been major blood loss or in animals with severe non-regenerative anaemia. Check the PCV to evaluate the need for blood. If it falls below 12–15%, the animal may need a transfusion, depending on speed of blood loss since chronic slow blood loss is tolerated better than sudden haemorrhage. Ferrets have no detectable blood groups, and there is little risk of a transfusion reaction. Collect blood from donor animals (preferably large males) into acid-citrate dextrose (ACD) anticoagulant, 1 ml ACD per 6 ml blood, and administer 6–12 ml at once to the recipient. The blood can be taken into heparin as an alternative.

Analgesia will be required after most surgical procedures, and will be most effective if given before the pain is perceived. Analgesics can be given as part of the premed, or after surgery before consciousness is regained. Always assess the level of pain or distress the animal is in before and after administering the analgesic to ensure it is having the desired effect. Doses of suitable analgesics are given in Table 18.4.

Table 18.4   Use of analgesics in ferrets.

Drug	Dose	Comments
Buprenorphine	0.05 mg/kg s.c. or i.m.	Lasts up to 12 hours.
Butorphanol	0.25 mg/kg s.c.	
Flunixin	0.5–2.0 mg/kg s.c.	
Ketoprofen	2 mg/kg s.c.	Administer once daily.
Aspirin	200 mg/kg p.o.	

It is important that the animal's appetite returns to normal following illness or surgery. Anorexic animals may need to be force fed using meat based baby foods or meat based convalescent diets for dogs and cats such as Hills canine/feline a/d, 2–5 ml three to four times daily. Nutri-plus gel (Virbac) may be given as a supplement in animals with a poor appetite.

If antibiotic therapy is required post-operatively, prolonged treatment should be by subcutaneous or oral administration, not intramuscular due to ferrets' small muscle mass.

19 COMMON SURGICAL PROCEDURES

Ferrets may be presented for any number of common surgical procedures, needing wounds to be sutured or neoplasms to be removed. The principles of surgery apply to all species, so approach any surgical procedure as for a cat or dog. Ferrets however are keen suture chewers, and will be very unforgiving if the sutures are uncomfortable. It is important to make sure that any wound is closed using appropriate suture materials and patterns. Subcuticular sutures using fine synthetic absorbable suture materials such as polyglactin 910 (Coated VICRYL®, Ethicon) are recommended for use in the skin.

Ferrets have a thick subcuticular layer, with the abdominal muscles being rather thin. The linea alba is well defined. Within the abdominal cavity, there is often a considerable quantity of fat which may obscure the abdominal organs. There is no caecum and the ileocolic junction is indistinguishable grossly as described in Chapter 1, but otherwise the abdominal anatomy is similar to the cat or dog. Particular care should be taken with cranial laparotomies, since the long thorax renders inadvertent penetration of the diaphragm and entry into the thoracic cavity during surgery a possibility, resulting in a life threatening pneumothorax.

Following abdominal surgery, ferrets appear to be prone to developing a serosanguinous discharge from the wound, particularly after long procedures or surgery for adrenal or pancreatic problems. The cause is unknown, and provided there is no infection or haemorrhage, the condition is self limiting and no treatment is required.

Ovariohysterectomy

Females which are not intended for breeding should ideally be spayed at six to eight months to prevent persistent oestrus and the concomitant health problems. This is best performed before the first oestrus, but can be carried out within one month of the onset of vulval swelling without post operative complications. Early neutering (at five to six weeks of age) may be associated with endocrine abnormalities and neoplasia (see Chapter 15). Animals which present when in oestrus should be spayed when out of oestrus: use hormone treatments (proligestone or human chorionic gonadotrophin) to induce ovulation (see Chapter 9). Prior to surgery on such animals, a blood sample should be taken to evaluate red cell and platelet numbers and morphology, to ensure that the animal is not anaemic and that blood clotting times are normal.

Spaying may also need to be carried out as a treatment for pyometra. This usually presents as a purulent vaginal discharge: polydipsia and polyuria are unusual. The technique is the same as for routine ovariohysterectomy, but particular care must be taken not to spill uterine contents into the abdominal cavity.

Female ferrets can be spayed using a ventral midline incision as for the bitch. An incision 4 cm in length over the midpoint between umbilicus and pubis should ensure adequate visibility. The uterus has two horns and is approximately 4 cm long. The ovaries lie caudal to the kidneys, concealed by a fat pad. The ovarian suspensory ligament is slack and may be torn easily. Double ligation if possible of the ovarian pedicle using a suitable absorbable suture material should be followed by a careful check to ensure all ovarian material has been included, otherwise the jill will have recurrent problems with persistent oestrus. A transfixion ligature across the anterior vagina will prevent ligature slippage and haemorrhage from the uterine arteries.

The incision can be closed using fine synthetic absorbable material such as 1.5 or 2 m polyglactin 910 (Coated VICRYL®, Ethicon). Use a simple interrupted pattern in the body wall, with a subcuticular suture in the skin.

Ovarian remnant surgery

If ovarian tissue is left behind after ovariohysterectomy, the jill will come into oestrus as normal and may develop hyperoestrogenism. Vulval swelling in a young spayed jill (one to two years) is most likely to be due to an ovarian remnant, whereas in older jills (over two years), adrenal tumours may produce the same effect. The two conditions may be differentiated by giving 0.5 ml proligestone s.c. or 100 i.u. human chorionic gonadotrophin i.m., which will cause the swelling to regress if due to an ovarian remnant, but not if due to an adrenal tumour.

Prior to exploratory surgery to remove the remnant, perform a complete blood count to ensure there is no platelet or red cell abnormality which could produce complications during and after surgery. A ventral midline incision extending slightly further cranially than for ovariohysterectomy will provide sufficient visibility to locate the remnant. These are usually to be found in the normal location caudolateral to the kidneys, although a remnant dropped during surgery may have implanted anywhere within the abdomen. Ligate the ovarian pedicle prior to removal of the ovary, and always check for a second remnant on the other side. The vulval swelling should regress within five days of surgery.

Castration

Castration may be done to reduce aggression between males, and can reduce the characteristic musky odour. Uni- or bilateral orchidectomy may be required in cases of malignancy. Castrated males are known as hobbles. Castration may be carried out using either scrotal incisions, as in the cat, or a closed prescrotal approach may be used as in the dog. The latter is preferable particularly out of the breeding season when the testicles are in a suprascrotal position. Clip and prepare the skin over the ventral caudal abdomen for surgery. Push one testicle up into a suprascrotal position, and incise through the skin overlying it. Remove the testicle within the tunica albuginea, ligating the spermatic cord tightly, then remove the other testicle through the same incision. Close the fascial layer with 1.5 m polyglactin 910, then use a subcuticular suture to close the skin.

Scrotal castration may be performed open or closed. The open 'self-tie' method is not suitable however, as the spermatic cord and vessels are too fragile to tie together, and these should be ligated using absorbable suture material.

Vasectomy

Vasectomised hobs may be needed to run with intact females to induce ovulation followed by pseudopregnancy, to prevent persistent oestrus. This is best performed when the hob is in season. The caudal abdomen is clipped and prepared for surgery, and two incisions are made in the skin either side of the midline, 3 cm cranial to the testes (see Plate 19). The vasa deferentia are small and a dissecting microscope or magnifying lens may be required to identify them. The spermatic cords can be found by blunt dissection, and the vasa deferentia separated. They should be double ligated using fine suture material (such as 1.5 metric polyglactin 910), and a portion of the vas removed between the ligatures. Alternatively, the animal may be vasectomised through a caudal midline laparotomy. The vasa deferentia may be identified and ligated as they loop over from the inguinal canal to enter the urethra at the bladder neck.

If there is any doubt about the procedure, the removed tissue can be sent for histology to confirm the vasectomy has been carried out correctly. Hobs cannot be assumed to be sterile until seven weeks after surgery.

Foreign body removal

Animals presenting with anorexia, lethargy, pawing at the mouth (due to nausea) or vomiting frequently have a gastric or intestinal foreign body, which may be palpable or visible on x-ray. Rubber or plastic objects are common, but fabric foreign bodies are also recorded, and contrast radiography may be required to locate radiolucent objects. If the clinical examination shows the animal to be dehydrated, stabilise it before surgery, but remove the object by routine gastrotomy or enterotomy as soon as possible after locating it.

Examine the entire gastro-intestinal tract for foreign bodies, since it is common for there to be more than one. At the same time, examine the liver, spleen and pancreas carefully, taking a biopsy of any abnormal tissue. It is not uncommon for animals to have concurrent *Helicobacter mustelae* infection, so a stomach wall biopsy from the pyloric area may be useful. Perform a gastrotomy, enterotomy or resection and anastomosis as for the cat or dog, remembering that ferrets' intestines are thin and friable, and great care must be taken to avoid tearing or strictures. Close incisions in the stomach in two layers, and intestinal incisions with a single layer using a fine (1–1.5 metric), preferably monofilament suture such as poliglecaprone 25 (Monocryl®, Ethicon) and a round bodied needle. Flush the abdominal cavity thoroughly with warmed sterile saline prior to closure to reduce contamination with gut contents. After surgery, maintain the animal on intravenous fluids for 12–24 hours, with nothing given by mouth. Soft foods can be given from 24 hours post operatively, and the animal can usually be discharged within 48 hours. Broad spectrum antibiotic cover should be started prior to surgery and continued until recovery is underway.

Adrenal gland surgery

Neoplasia of the adrenal glands is commonly reported in ferrets in North America, often in females, and surgery is the only definitive treatment. The disease may be bilateral, or associated with concurrent pancreatic insulinoma or paraurethral cysts (see below), so a ventral midline approach is best. The adrenal glands can be located by palpation in the fat pads craniomedial to the kidneys. They are usually pink in colour, 6–8 mm long and 2–3 mm thick, and have the texture of a cooked lentil. Any enlargement or increase in firmness indicates abnormality.

Removal of the left gland is easier than the right, which is further cranial, lies beneath the right lobe of the liver and is often adherent to the caudal vena cava. The left gland can be dissected away from the fat, carefully ligating any minor vessels. There may be considerable haemorrhage or ooze from vessels in the fat, and the application of haemostatic dressings may be useful, (e.g. Kaltostat®, ConvaTec). Large tumours may extend towards the midline, and care must be taken not to interrupt the mesenteric blood supply. Removal of the right gland may be achieved by incising the capsule and 'shelling out' the glandular tissue, since removal of the capsule almost invariably results in damage to the vena cava. If removal of the capsule is required, the vena cava can be ligated longitudinally using a haemostatic clip where the adrenal gland is attached to prevent haemorrhage when the gland is removed. See Mullen (1997) for a more detailed description of adrenal gland surgery. Clinical signs usually regress shortly after adrenalectomy. Vulval swelling will subside within one to two weeks, and hair regrowth occurs after two to eight weeks.

Other common procedures

Ferrets in North America are reportedly prone to pancreatic insulinomas, and debulking of tumour tissue can render medical management more successful (see Chapter 9). Ferrets undergoing surgery for insulinomas should be given 5% dextrose solution intravenously to prevent hypoglycaemia during the procedure, and be starved for several hours prior to surgery. Using a cranial ventral midline laparotomy incision, palpate the pancreas to locate any nodules, but handle it carefully to avoid causing pancreatitis. Insulinomas are found as multiple, red brown well defined masses 2 mm to 1 cm across, which will 'shell out' using blunt dissection. Haemorrhage can be controlled using haemostatic dressings. Check the liver and spleen for metastatic nodules, and check the adrenals at the same time since adrenal tumours are often found in animals with insulinomas. Prior to closure of the incision, lavage the pancreas and abdominal cavity copiously with sterile saline to flush out any pancreatic enzymes. Following removal of the tumours, maintain the animal on a 5% dextrose drip and withhold food and water for

12 hours to reduce pancreatic secretions. Check the blood glucose level every 6–12 hours: this should rise quickly. Once this is apparent and the animal is feeding (12 hours or so after surgery), the dextrose drip may be stopped.

Male animals with adrenal tumours may present with stranguria, found to be due to a cystic mass surrounding the bladder neck. These are known as paraurethral or prostatic cysts, although the ferret has little distinguishable prostate tissue. These masses are partly cystic and partly solid, and may occasionally communicate with the urethra. The origin of these masses is unknown although they may be caused by cystic hypertrophy of the prostatic tissue. They usually regress spontaneously after adrenalectomy.

Reference

Mullen, H. (1997) Soft tissue surgery. In: E.V. Hillyer and K.H. Quesenberry (eds). *Ferrets, Rabbits and Rodents: Clinical Medicine and Surgery.* W.B. Saunders Company, Philadelphia, pp. 131–44.

Further reading

Chapter 16

Besch-Williford, C.L. (1987) Biology and medicine of the ferret. *Veterinary Clinics of North America: Small Animal Practice*, **17**, pp. 1155–83.

Brown, S.A. (1998) Clinical pathology of small mammals. Paper given to BSAVA Congress, Birmingham, UK.

Douglas, S.W., Herrtage, M.E. and Williamson, H.D. (1987) *Principles of Veterinary Radiography*. 4th edn. Baillière Tindall, London.

Moody, K.D., Bowman, T.A. and Lang, C.M. (1985) Laboratory management of the ferret for biomedical research. *Laboratory Animal Science*, **35**(3), pp. 272–9.

Porter, V. and Brown, N. (1997) *The Complete Book of Ferrets*. D & M Publications, Bedford.

Quesenberry, K.E. (1997) Basic approach to veterinary care. In: E.V. Hillyer and K.H. Quesenberry (eds). *Ferrets, Rabbits and Rodents: Clinical Medicine and Surgery*. W.B. Saunders, Philadelphia, pp. 14–25.

Rosenthal, K. (1994) Ferrets. *Veterinary Clinics of North America: Small Animal Practice*, **24**, pp. 1–23.

Wolfensohn, S.E. and Lloyd, M.H. (1998) *A Handbook of Laboratory Animal Management and Welfare*. Blackwell Science, Oxford.

Wolvekamp, P. (1998) Radiography of small mammals: techniques and interpretation. Paper given to BSAVA Congress, Birmingham, UK.

Chapter 17

Besch-Williford, C.L. (1987) Biology and medicine of the ferret. *Veterinary Clinics of North America: Small Animal Practice*, **17**, pp. 1155–83.

Bleakley, S.P. (1980) Simple technique for bleeding ferrets. *Laboratory Animals*, **14**, pp. 59–60.

Brown, S.A. (1998) Clinical pathology of small mammals. Paper given to BSAVA Congress, Birmingham, UK.

Fox, J.G. (1998) Normal clinical and biological parameters. In: J.G. Fox (ed.). *Biology and Diseases of the Ferret*. 2nd edn. Williams and Wilkins, Baltimore, pp. 183–210.

Hem, A., Smith, A.J. and Solberg, P. (1998) Saphenous venepuncture for blood sampling of the mouse, rat, hamster, gerbil, guinea pig, ferret and mink. *Laboratory Animals*, **32**, pp. 364–8.

Howard, J. (1993) Semen collection and analysis in carnivores. In: M.E. Fowler (ed.), *Zoo and Wild Animal Medicine: Current Therapy 3*. W.B. Saunders, Philadelphia, pp. 390–8.

Marini, R.P., Esteves, M.I. and Fox, J.G. (1994) A technique for catheterization of the urinary bladder in the ferret. *Laboratory Animals*, **28**, pp. 155–7.

Otto, G., Rosenblad, W.D. and Fox, J.G. (1993) Practical venepuncture techniques for the ferret. *Laboratory Animals*, **27**, pp. 26–9.

Palley, L.S., Marini, R.P., Rosenblad, W.D. and Fox, J.G. (1990) A technique for femoral bone marrow collection in the ferret. *Laboratory Animal Science*, **40**, pp. 654–5.

Quesenberry, K.E. (1997) Basic approach to veterinary care. In: E.V. Hillyer and K.H. Quesenberry (eds). *Ferrets, Rabbits and Rodents: Clinical Medicine and Surgery*. W.B. Saunders, Philadelphia, pp. 14–25.

Chapter 18

Besch-Williford, C.L. (1987) Biology and medicine of the ferret. *Veterinary Clinics of North America: Small Animal Practice*, **17**, pp. 1155–83.

Flecknell, P.A. (1997) *Laboratory Animal Anaesthesia*. 2nd edn. Academic Press, London.

Hall, L.W. and Clarke, K.W. (1991) *Veterinary Anaesthesia*. 7th edn. Baillière Tindall, London.

Manning, D.D. and Bell, J.A. (1990) Lack of detectable blood groups in domestic ferrets: implications for transfusion. *Journal of the American Veterinary Medical Association*, **197**, pp. 84–6.

Marini, R.P. and Fox, J.G. (1998) Anaesthesia, surgery and biomethodology. In: J.G. Fox (ed.). *Biology and Diseases of the Ferret*. 2nd edn. Williams and Wilkins, Baltimore, pp. 449–84.

Moody, K.D., Bowman, T.A. and Lang, C.M. (1985) Laboratory management of the ferret for biomedical research. *Laboratory Animal Science*, **35**(3), pp. 272–9.

Quesenberry, K.E. (1997) Basic approach to veterinary care. In: E.V.

Hillyer and K.H. Quesenberry (eds). *Ferrets, Rabbits and Rodents: Clinical Medicine and Surgery.* W.B. Saunders, Philadelphia, pp. 14–25.

Wolfensohn S.E. and Lloyd M.H. (1998) *A Handbook of Laboratory Animal Management and Welfare.* Blackwell Science, Oxford.

Chapter 19

Besch-Williford, C.L. (1987) Biology and medicine of the ferret. *Veterinary Clinics of North America: Small Animal Practice*, **17**, pp. 1155–83.

Burke, T.J. (1988) Common diseases and medical management of ferrets. In: E.R. Jacobson and G.V. Kollias (eds). *Exotic Animals.* Churchill Livingstone, Edinburgh, pp. 247–60.

Lumeij, J.T., van der Hage, M.H., Dorrestein, G.M. and van Sluis, F.J. (1987) Hypoglycaemia due to a functional pancreatic islet cell tumour (insulinoma) in a ferret (*Mustela putorius furo*). *Veterinary Record*, **120**, p. 129.

Marini, R.P. and Fox, J.G. (1998) Anaesthesia, surgery and biomethodology. In: J.G. Fox (ed.). *Biology and Diseases of the Ferret.* 2nd edn. Williams and Wilkins, Baltimore, pp. 449–84.

Mullen, H. (1997) Soft tissue surgery. In: E.V. Hillyer and K.H. Quesenberry (eds). *Ferrets, Rabbits and Rodents: Clinical Medicine and Surgery.* W.B. Saunders Company, Philadelphia, pp. 131–44.

Oxenham, M. (1991) Ferrets. In: P.H. Beynon and J.E. Cooper (eds). *Manual of Exotic Pets.* British Small Animal Veterinary Association, Cheltenham.

SECTION 4
USEFUL INFORMATION

20 BIOLOGICAL DATA

Biological parameters are often used for the routine assessment of an animal's state of health or disease. Knowledge of normal values is essential in the interpretation of any results.

Haematology

Assessment of the blood profile is essential in the diagnostic workup of many ferret diseases. Little data has been published on normal values for haematology in ferrets, although three studies performed on ferrets in Britain and the USA showed them to have similar values to the cat, except for a higher red cell count and haemoglobin level, and a higher percentage of reticulocytes. Blood may be collected relatively easily from conscious ferrets if they are used to handling, but if not then sedation or anaesthesia may be required. This can alter the results, e.g. isoflurane produces a fall in packed cell volume, haemoglobin level and red cell count, possibly due to sequestering of cells in the spleen, so results must be interpreted with care, in conjunction with an assessment of the clinical signs and history. Ferret-specific factors should be taken into account as well, for example, a rise in white cell count is more often an indicator of neoplasia than infection. A small increase in the erythrocyte and neutrophil counts and reduction in lymphocyte level may be noticed with increasing age. The normal packed cell volume in ferrets is between 40–60%, and they have a reduced erythrocyte sedimentation rate, so samples need to be centrifuged for 20% longer

Table 20.1   Normal data.

Biological Data		Breeding Data	
Adult weight male (grams)[a]	1000–2000	Puberty (months)	8–12
Adult weight female (grams)[a]	600–950	Age to breed male (days)	from 275–365
Food intake (grams)[b]	50–75	Age to breed female (days)	275
Water intake (ml)	75–100	Gestation (days)	38–44
Lifespan (years)	5–9		Average 42
Rectal temperature (°C)	37.8–40.0	Litter size	2–17 (average 8)
Heart rate/min.	160–320	Birth weight (grams)	6–12
Blood pressure systole (mm Hg)	140 ± 35	Eyes open (days)	34
Blood pressure diastole (mm Hg)	110 ± 31	Onset of hearing (days)	32
Respiratory rate/min.	33–36	Weaning age (weeks)	6–7
Diploid number	40	Oestrous cycle	Induced ovulator, cycle determined by day length

[a] Both sexes show a periodic weight fluctuation of 30–40%. Fat is laid down in autumn and lost in winter.
[b] Dry carnivore pelleted diet. This should be fed soaked in hot water to form a paste for ferrets – give 140–190 g daily.

Table 20.2   Haematological data.

	Albino		Fitch	
	Male	*Female*	*Male*	*Female*
RBC ($\times 10^6$/mm^3)	7.3–12.18	6.77–9.76	9.7–13.2	9.7–13.2
PCV (%)	44–61	42–55	36–50	47–51
Hb (g/dl)	16.3–18.2	14.8–17.4	12.0–16.3	15.2–17.4
Platelets ($\times 10^3$/mm^3)	297–730	310–910		
Reticulocytes (%)	1–12	2–14		
WBC ($\times 10^3$/mm^3)	4.4–19.1	4.0–18.2	5.6–10.8	2.5–8.6
Neutrophils (%)	11–82	43–84	24–78	12–41
Lymphocytes (%)	12–54	12–50	28–69	25–95
Eosinophils (%)	0–7	0–5	0–7	1–9
Monocytes (%)	0–9	208	3.4–8.2	1.7–6.3
Basophils (%)	0–2	0–1	0–2.7	0–2.9

A prothrombin time of 14.4–16.5 seconds has been recorded.

than for other species in order to determine the packed cell volume and to obtain serum samples.

Biochemistry

The high packed cell volume of ferrets means that samples for biochemistry need to be relatively large. Take three times the volume of blood as the amount of plasma or serum required. Serum chemistry values for ferrets seem to be similar to those in dogs and cats, and like these species there is an age related decrease in the alkaline phosphatase level. High levels of liver enzymes are often associated with Aleutian disease virus infection, so this should be ruled out in these cases.

Urinalysis

When taking samples for urinalysis, ensure the sample is fresh and refrigerate it if necessary. For microbiology, collect a large sterile sample and centrifuge it, then use the sediment for culture. Samples may be collected by cystocentesis, catheterisation or from the floor as they are voided naturally (see Chapter 17). Normal ferret urine is yellow in colour and can have a pungent odour. Trace amounts of

Table 20.3 Biochemical data.

	Albino	Fitch (Polecat)
Serum protein (g/dl)	5.1–7.4	5.3–7.2
Albumin (g/dl)	2.6–3.8	3.3–4.1
Globulin (g/dl)	2.5–4.8	
Glucose (mg/dl)	94–207	62.5–134
Blood urea nitrogen (mg/dl)	10–45	12–43
Creatinine (mg/dl)	0.4–0.9	0.2–0.6
Total bilirubin (mg/dl)	< 1	0–0.1
Cholesterol (mg/dl)	64–296	119–209
Sodium (mmol/l)	137–162	146–160
Potassium (mmol/l)	4.5–7.7	4.3–5.3
Calcium (mg/dl)	8.0–11.8	8.6–10.5
Phosphorus (mg/dl)	4.0–9.1	5.6–8.7
Alanine aminotransferase (U/l)		82–289
Aspartate aminotransferase (U/l)	28–120	57–248
Alkaline phosphatase (U/l)	9–84	30–120

protein are common (Table 20.4), and blood may be present in the urine of oestrous females with no ill effect.

Special diagnostic tests: hormone evaluations

Hormone levels may need to be determined in cases of endocrine or reproductive disorders, adrenal neoplasia, or pancreatic insulinoma. Normal values for many hormones are given in Table 20.5.

Reproductive hormones

Evaluation of these is important in the assessment of adrenal-related endocrinopathy. The levels of all hormones may rise significantly in these cases.

Table 20.4 Normal values for urinalysis.

	Male	Female
Volume produced in 24 hours (ml)	8–48	8–140
pH	6.5–7.5	6.5–7.5
Protein (mg/dl)	7–33	0–32
Ketones	+	+

Table 20.5 Hormone levels.

Hormone	Male	Female
Androstenedione (nmol/l)	6.6	
Dehydroepiandrosterone sulphate (μmol/l)	0.01	
Oestradiol (pmol/l)	106	
17-hydroxyprogesterone (nmol/l)	0.4	
Cortisol (μg/dl)	0.22–2.7	0.55–1.84
T3 (ng/ml)	0.45–0.78	0.29–0.73
T4 (μg/dl)	1.01–8.29	0.7–3.43
Insulin (pmol/l)	35–250	

Cortisol

Signs of Cushing's disease are rare in ferrets, but evaluation of cortisol may be required. To properly evaluate adrenal function, an ACTH stimulation test may be needed. Give 1 unit/kg of ACTH i.m.: this should produce an increase of 40% in the cortisol level within 30–60 minutes. The low dose dexamethasone suppression test can be used to determine if the cause is pituitary or adrenal. Administer 0.1 mg/kg dexamethasone i.m. or i.v.. The cortisol level should decrease by 27% six hours post injection. In cases of hyperadrenocorticism, the fall is much less. In pituitary dependent hyperadrenocorticism, there may be some suppression at four hours with a return to normal at eight hours. In both these diagnostic tests, a more dramatic result which may be easier to interpret is obtained if the drugs are given i.v.

Thyroid hormones

Some disorders of thyroid function have been reported in ferrets. Plasmacytic, lymphocytic thyroiditis may occur with Aleutian disease virus, thyroid adenomas have been reported, and thyroid dysfunction may be associated with alopecia or other dermatologic disorders. Thyroid function testing can be useful in these cases. Adult entire male ferrets have higher levels of T_4 than females, juveniles or castrated males.

Thyroid function can be evaluated by the intravenous administration of 1 I.U. TSH. There should be a significant rise in T_4 level at one, two and six hours post injection compared with a baseline sample.

Insulin

Evaluation of insulin levels may be useful in the diagnosis of insulinoma.

Further reading

Andrews, P.L.R., Bower, A.J. and Illman, O. (1979) Some aspects of the physiology and anatomy of the cardiovascular system of the ferret, *Mustela putorius furo. Laboratory Animals*, **13**, pp. 215–20.

Besch-Williford, C.L. (1987) Biology and medicine of the ferret. *Veterinary Clinics of North America: Small Animal Practice*, **17**, pp. 1155–83.

Brown, S.A. (1998) Clinical pathology. Paper given to BSAVA Congress, Birmingham.

Fox, J.G. *et al.* (1986) Serum chemistry and haematology reference values in the ferret (*Mustela putorius furo*). *Laboratory Animal Science*, **36**, p. 583.

Fox, J.G. (1998) Normal clinical and biologic parameters. In: J.G. Fox (ed.). *Biology and Diseases of the Ferret*. 2nd edn. Williams and Wilkins, Baltimore, pp. 183–210.

Garibaldi, B.A., Pecquet-Goad, M.E. and Fox, J.G. (1987) Serum cortisol radioimmunoassay values in the normal ferret and response to ACTH stimulation and dexamethasone suppression tests. *Laboratory Animal Science*, **37**, p. 545.

Garibaldi, B.A., Pecquet-Goad, M.E. and Fox, J.G. (1987) Serum thyroxine (T_4) and tri-iodothyronine (T_3) radioimmunoassay values in the normal ferret. *Laboratory Animal Science*, **37**, p. 544.

Lee, E.J., Moore, W.E., Fryer, H.C. and Minocha, H.C. (1982) Haematological and serum chemistry profiles of ferrets (*Mustela putorius furo*). *Laboratory Animals*, **16**, pp. 133–7.

McKellar, Q.A. (1989) Drug dosages for small mammals. *In Practice*, **11**, pp. 57–61.

Morrisey, J.K. (1997) Differential diagnoses for clinical problems in ferrets. In: E.V. Hillyer and K.H. Quesenberry (eds). *Ferrets, Rabbits and Rodents: Clinical Medicine and Surgery*. W.B. Saunders, Philadelphia, pp. 405–7.

Quesenberry, K.E. (1997) Basic approach to veterinary care. In: E.V. Hillyer and K.H. Quesenberry (eds). *Ferrets, Rabbits and Rodents: Clinical Medicine and Surgery*. W.B. Saunders, Philadelphia, pp. 14–25.

Porter, V. and Brown, N. (1997) *The Complete Book of Ferrets*. D & M Publications, Bedford.

Rosenthal, K. (1994) Ferrets. *Veterinary Clinics of North America: Small Animal Practice*, **24**, pp. 1–23.

Rosenthal, K.L. and Quesenberry, K.E. (1997) Endocrine diseases. In: E.V. Hillyer and K.E. Quesenberry (eds). *Ferrets, Rabbits, and Rodents: Clinical Medicine and Surgery*. W.B. Saunders, Philadelphia, pp. 85–98.

Smith, D.A. and Burgmann, P.M. (1997) Formulary. In: E.V. Hillyer and K.E. Quesenberry (eds). *Ferrets, Rabbits, and Rodents: Clinical Medicine and Surgery*. W.B. Saunders, Philadelphia, pp. 392–403.

Thornton, P.C., Wright, P.A., Sacra, P.J. and Goodier, T.E.W. (1979) The ferret, *Mustela putorius furo*, as a new species in toxicology. *Laboratory Animals*, **13**, p. 119.

APPENDIX 1: DIFFERENTIAL DIAGNOSES FOR COMMON PRESENTING SIGNS

Abdominal mass	GI foreign body
	Neoplasia, e.g. ovarian, adrenal
	Mesenteric lymph node enlargement
	Polycystic kidneys/ hydronephrosis
	Splenomegaly
	Urinary tract obstruction
Alopecia	Adrenal related endocrinopathy
	Fungal infection
	External parasites
	Hyperoestrogenism
	Mast cell tumour
	Nutritional deficiency
	Ovarian neoplasia
	Seasonal variation
Anaemia	Aleutian disease
	Bone marrow neoplasia
	Chronic disease of any nature
	Flea infestation
	Gastrointestinal ulceration
	Haemorrhage
	Hyperoestrogenism
	Thrombocytopenia
	Zinc toxicity
Ascites	Abdominal neoplasia
	Cardiac disease

Ataxia/weakness	Aleutian disease
	Botulism
	Cardiac disease
	CNS trauma, neoplasia, infection
	Hyperoestrogenism
	Hypocalcaemia
	Insulinoma – hypoglycaemia
	Intervertebral disc disease
	Lymphosarcoma
	Metabolic disease
	Osteodystrophy
	Posterior paresis
	Septicaemia
	Spinal injury
	Thiamine deficiency
	Viral myelitis
	Zinc deficiency
Cervical swelling	Abscess
	Actinomyces
	Foreign body
	Haematoma
	Neoplasia
	Salivary mucocoele
Chronic wasting	Aleutian disease
	Chronic GI foreign body
	Chronic nephritis
	Dental disease
	Gastroenteritis
	Hyperoestrogenism
	Internal parasites
	Megaoesophagus
	Neoplasia
	Proliferative bowel disease
Diarrhoea	Dietary intolerance
	Gastroenteritis (includes *Salmonella*, *Campylobacter*, rotavirus, eosinophilic gastroenteritis, epizootic catarrhal enteritis)

GI foreign body
Internal parasites
Proliferative bowel disease
Systemic infection

Dysuria   Paraurethral/prostatic cyst (male)
                               Urinary tract disease/uroliths

Hypersalivation/ptyalism   Botulism
                               Canine distemper virus
                               Dental disease
                               Gastroenteritis
                               GI foreign body
                               Hypoglycaemia

Neurological signs   Addison's disease
                               Aleutian disease
                               Botulism
                               Canine distemper virus
                               Insulinoma – hypoglycaemia
                               Non-specific encephalitis
                               Toxins
                               Toxoplasmosis
                               Trauma

Ocular discharge/   Canine distemper virus
conjunctivitis   Ophthalmia neonatorum (kits)
                               Salmonella

Pruritus   Adrenal related endocrinopathy
                               Dermatitis
                               External parasites
                               Fungal infection
                               Mast cell tumour

Respiratory signs   Canine distemper virus
                               Cardiomyopathy/cardiac disease
                               Influenza virus
                               Intrathoracic mass
                               Ketoacidosis
                               Malignant hyperthermia

	Neoplasia
	Pleural effusion or transudate
	Pneumonia
	Ruptured diaphragm
Seizures	Canine distemper virus
	CNS infection
	CNS neoplasia
	CNS trauma
	Hypocalcaemia
	Insulinoma – hypoglycaemia
	Toxaemia
Skin lesions	*Actinomyces*
	Canine distemper
	External parasites
	Fungal infection
	Neoplasia
	Trauma
Splenomegaly	Incidental finding in 'normal animals'
	Lymphoma
	Primary splenic disease, e.g. haemangioma
Sudden death	Anthrax
	Botulism
	Gastric haemorrhage
	Toxaemia, e.g. pyometra
Tarry stools/melaena	Aleutian disease virus
	Gastric ulcers
	GI foreign body
	Helicobacter mustelae
	Hyperoestrogenism
	Pregnancy toxaemia
Vomiting/regurgitation	Gastroenteritis
	GI foreign body
	GI neoplasia
	Helicobacter mustelae
	Insulinoma

Megaoesophagus
Metabolic disease
Oesophageal foreign body

Vulval swelling   Adrenal related endocrinopathy
Hyperoestrogenism
Oestrus
Ovarian neoplasia
Ovarian remnant
Vaginitis

APPENDIX 2: DRUG DOSES FOR USE IN FERRETS

Antimicrobials	Dose	Route
Amoxycillin	10–20 mg/kg b.i.d	p.o., s.c.
Ampicillin	5–10 mg/kg b.i.d	s.c., i.m., i.v.
Cephalexin	15–25 mg/kg b.i.d or t.i.d	p.o.
Chloramphenicol	50 mg/kg b.i.d	p.o., s.c., i.m.
Clavulanate-potentiated amoxycillin	10–20 mg/kg b.i.d	p.o., s.c.
Enrofloxacin	5–15 mg/kg b.i.d	p.o., s.c., i.m.
Erythromycin	10 mg/kg q.i.d	p.o.
Gentamicin	4–8 mg/kg in divided doses	s.c., i.m., i.v.
Lincomycin	10–15 mg/kg t.i.d	p.o.
	10 mg/kg b.i.d	i.m
Metronidazole	10–20 mg/kg	p.o.
Neomycin	10–20 mg/kg tid or q.i.d	p.o.
Oxytetracycline	20 mg/kg t.i.d	p.o.
Trimethoprim-sulpha combinations	15–30 mg/kg bid	p.o., s.c.
	30 mg/kg s.i.d for 2 weeks	p.o. (for coccidiosis)

Analgesics (see also Chapter 18)	Dose	Route
Aspirin	200 mg/kg b.i.d	p.o.
Buprenorphine	0.05 mg/kg b.i.d	s.c. or i.m.
Butorphanol	0.25 mg/kg	s.c.
Flunixin	0.5–2.0 mg/kg	s.c. no more than 3 days
Ketoprofen	2 mg/kg s.i.d	s.c.

Antiparasiticides

Fenbendazole 22% granules	0.5 g/kg	p.o.
Ivermectin	200–400 µg/kg Every 2–4 weeks until parasites eradicated	s.c.
Piperazine	50–100 mg/kg Repeat after 2 weeks	p.o.
Pyrethrin products	Topically once per week	

Antifungals

Griseofulvin	25 mg/kg s.i.d 3–6 weeks	p.o.

Other drugs

Dexamethasone	4–8 mg/kg once	i.m., i.v. for shock
Doxapram	5–11 mg/kg	i.v.
Enalapril	0.25–0.5 mg/kg daily or alternate days	p.o.
Frusemide	1–4 mg/kg b.i.d or t.i.d	i.m., i.v.
hCG	20–100 I.U. once	i.m.
Nandrolone	2–5 mg/kg, repeat as required	s.c.
Oxytocin	0.2–3.0 units/kg	s.c., i.m.
Prednisolone	0.5–2.5 mg/kg s.i.d or b.i.d	p.o.
Proligestone	0.5 ml/kg (50 mg/kg) once	s.c., i.m.

INDEX